Mind Maps of Clinical Research Basics

Mind Maps of Clinical Research Basics

by

Amrita Akhouri

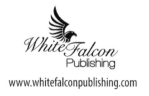

White Falcon Publishing

www.whitefalconpublishing.com

Mind Maps of Clinical Research Basics
Amrita Akhouri

www.whitefalconpublishing.com

ISBN - 978-93-87193-37-6

"Dedicated to my loving parents and most humbly to all my readers"

PREFACE

Thank you to all the readers for an excellent response to my book "Mind Maps of Pharmacovigilance Basics" which was published in the year 2015. Enthused by this response, I decided to write a book on Clinical Research on similar lines (explaining the subject through Mind Maps) and I am delighted to present this book to all of you.

There are many books available in the market on Clinical Research and those books provide great insights into the subject, however, the subject fundamentals become easy to understand if the concepts are presented in a manner which is interesting to read and easy to revise.

With 350 plus mind maps, short notes, glossary and the text contents, this book serves as a quick and easy reckoner.

The chapter on careers in clinical research gives an insight into the main job roles in the field of Clinical Research along with the focus on how to prepare for job interviews. Hence, this book will be very helpful to the students as well as to the job seekers trying to make a career in the field of clinical research.

I hope you enjoy reading this book.

If you wish to give any feedback/suggestions on this book, please feel free to write to me at aakhouri6@gmail.com or visit my website www.amritaakhouri.com

CONTENTS

4. CLINICAL RESEARCH – VARIOUS DESIGNS   **39**

17.   SHORT NOTES   286

Chapter 1

INTRODUCTION TO CLINICAL RESEARCH

1.1 Learnings from the chapter

- *Brief introduction to drug development process*
- *Definition of Clinical Research and details about different types, different players, scope, importance and outcomes of clinical research*
- *Outline of Biomedical Research*
- *Basic overview of scientific research*

1.2 Introduction

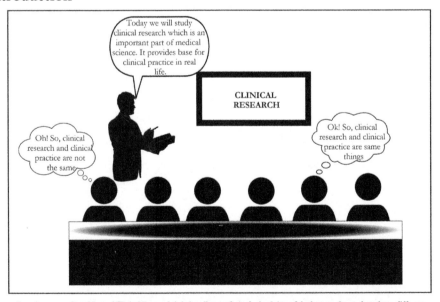

In a classroom, the subject of Clinical Research is being discussed. At the begining of the lecture, the students have different opinion on the subject. Some of them think that Clinical Research and Clinical Practice are same whereas some other students think that these two are different! But actually, these two are not same.

Clinical research and clinical practice are not the same. In fact, clinical research is the foundation of clinical practice.

In order to test new therapeutic products for their safety and efficacy, clinical research works under controlled conditions whereas, clinical practice works in the real-time environment and uses the products tested through clinical research.

Healthcare providers (e.g., physician, etc.) generally prescribe medicine that has received a hallmark of safety and effectiveness for usage among the general population (refer to the **Fig – Clinical research and clinical practice are different**). In the figure (Fig – Clinical research and clinical practice are different), drug X can be considered safe for human consumption because it has been studied and tested in humans in accordance with the required regulations.

Prior to introduction to the general population, any new medicinal product is studied in the laboratory setup and also on the animals in order to develop an understanding of the physiological and chemical properties of the product as well as its pharmacological effect and toxicology. Post animal studies, the investigational product is studied in humans to test and prove the safety and efficacy of the new entity.

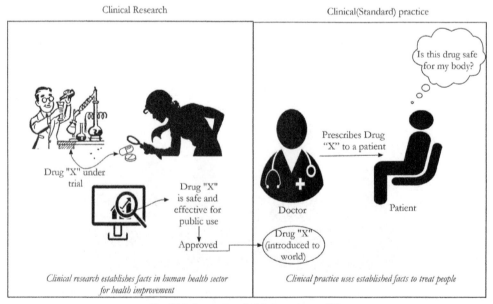

Fig: Clinical research and clinical practice are different

1.3 Drug Development Process - Overview

Understanding the disease and developing the appropriate (safe and effective) medicine is a long, arduous and expensive affair [refer to the **Fig – Disease to drug (time taken and cost to produce)**]. On an average it takes about 10 - 15 years to develop a drug from its discovery phase to getting it approved and making it available in the market for its usage.

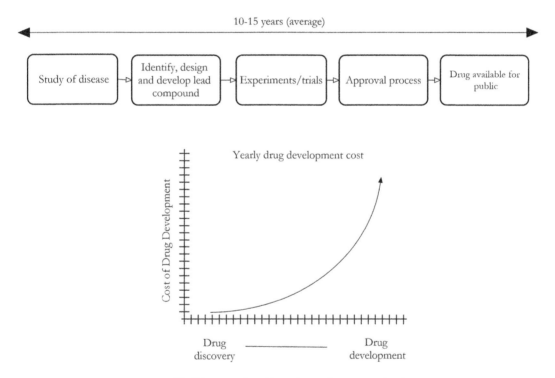

Fig: Disease to drug (time taken and cost to produce)

The generalized process of getting a new drug to the market [refer to the **Fig – Drug development process (summarized)**] involves the following steps:

- Discovery of a new potential compound (drug)

- Studies to be conducted in animals (pre-clinical research) to check the safety and efficacy of new potential compound

- Submission of Investigational New Drug Application (INDA) to the FDA

- Post INDA approval, the studies need to be conducted in humans i.e., clinical research has to be done in order to study the safety and efficacy of a new entity in human body. These studies generally occur in four phases which are as follows:

- Phase 1 Clinical trials (clinical trial is one of the types of clinical research) - intended to study the safety aspects and dosage of the investigational product

- Phase 2 clinical trials – intended to study the safety profile and efficacy of investigational product

- Phase 3 clinical trials – intended to gather more information in order to ascertain the safety and efficacy of the investigational product

- Submission of New Drug Application (NDA) to the FDA (for getting approval to introduce new entity in the market)

- Phase 4 trials - intended to study the effects of the new drug in wider population

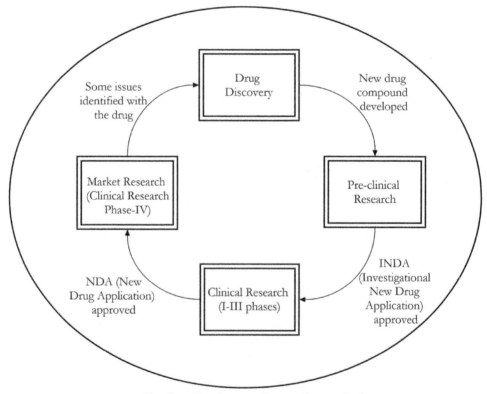

Fig: Drug Development Process (Summarized)

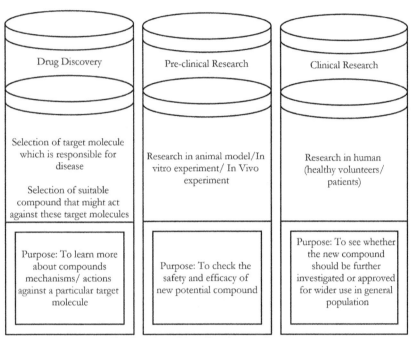

Fig: Overview of Drug Development Process

{Note: For details about drug discovery and pre-clinical research, please refer to the book - "Mind Maps of Pharmacovigilance Basics" by the same author.}

1.4 Clinical Research - Introduction

Clinical research is an exhaustive process of determining the safety and efficacy of a candidate product (vaccine, diagnostic, and therapeutic). Only those prospective compounds which have fared satisfactorily through the basic and the preclinical research phases are approved for clinical trials in humans, and a small number of those ones finally sail through the various phases and approvals involved in bringing the product to the market.

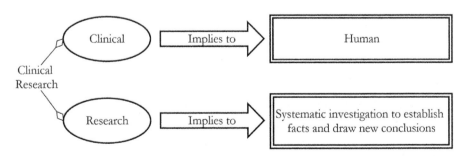

1.5 Definition of Clinical Research

Clinical research is a branch of healthcare science that determines the safety and effectiveness (efficacy) of medications, devices, diagnostic products and treatment regimens intended for human use. These may be used for prevention, treatment, diagnosis or for relieving symptoms of a disease.

Clinical research is an integral part of Biomedical research or we can say clinical research is the subset of Biomedical research.

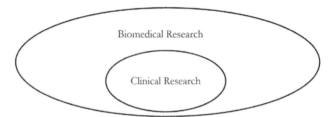

Fig: Clinical Research is the subset of Biomedical Research

1.6 Biomedical Research

Biomedical research is a complete set of research from the theoretical to practical application. Medical research works to unlock the basis of medical treatment by using a variety of approaches such as biology, chemistry, pharmacology and toxicology, etc.

In short, it can be viewed as encompassing basic research, preclinical research (e.g. in cellular systems and animal models) and clinical research (e.g. clinical trials) [refer to the **Fig – Biomedical Research**].

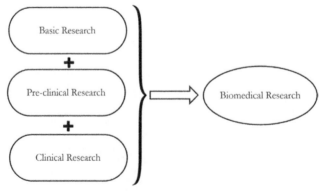

Fig: Biomedical Research

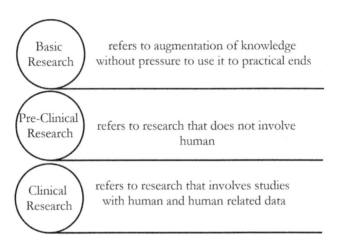

Fig: Summarized overview of Biomedical Research

1.7 Scientific Research – Basic Overview

A research question is the question which needs to be answered through the conduct of research (i.e., research question refers to "what does a researcher want to study?"). While, a hypothesis is "not a question", but rather it is a "statement" about the relationship between two or more variables.

Where do research questions come from?

There can be many reasons for the creation of a research question. Some of those reasons are mentioned in the **Fig – Reasons for origin of research question.**

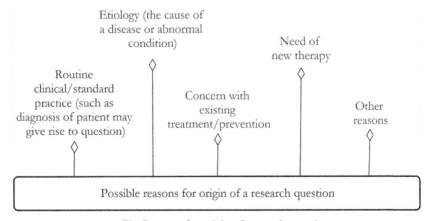

Fig: Reasons for origin of research question

Hypothesis is an assumption which explains the research question and its objectives in a focused way to aid the correct research conduct. A clear hypothesis tells about the relevant and irreverent aspects of a research (refer to the **Fig – Benefit of clearly stated hypothesis**).

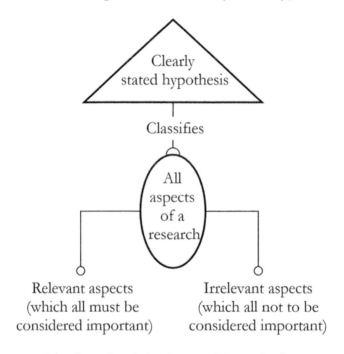

Fig: Benefit of clearly stated hypothesis

Thus, the hypothesis supports in deciding which all variables have to be manipulated or measured, which population has to be examined, the proposed outcome for the research, etc. A researcher formulates research hypotheses (i.e., null hypothesis and research hypothesis) to answer a research question (refer to the **Fig – Null hypothesis and research hypothesis**).

In an effort to disapprove a null hypothesis, the researcher creates an alternative hypothesis. Thus, arises the need to do a research intended to approve/disapprove a null hypothesis or alternative hypothesis and ultimately answer the research question. This process needs a well-designed research plan which must contain all the required stuff (such as methodology, study duration, types of samples required, data collection techniques, data analysis, result interpretation, etc.) in order to conduct a study (refer to the **Fig – Scientific research - Basic overview**). The facts and information obtained from this study establishes new clinical evidences for clinical practices which in turn leads to the new research question for future study.

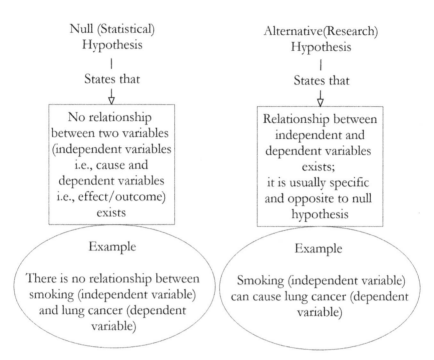

Fig: Null hypothesis and Alternative hypothesis

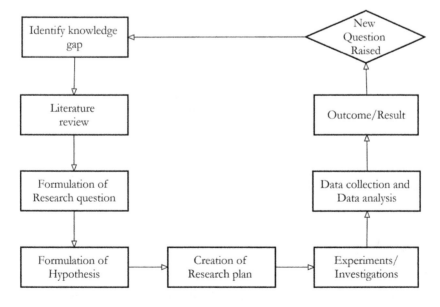

Fig: Scientific Research - Basic Overview

Results from clinical research contribute to the development of new drugs, new treatment procedures and new tools. Additionally, it also spurs new research questions for further research which gives birth to new discoveries over a period of time and helps us to understand the diseases better (refer to the **Fig- Translation of Basic Research into Clinical practice**).

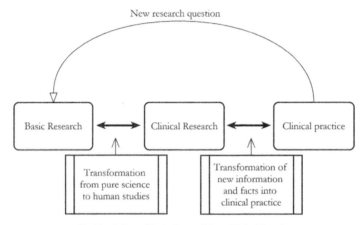

Fig: Tanslation of Basic Research into Clinical Practice

1.8 Important players in Clinical Research

Clinical research is a vast field. Hence, it involves a number of people with different roles and responsibilities whose combined efforts brings out the results of a research. Few important players are mentioned in the **Fig – Important players in a clinical research.**

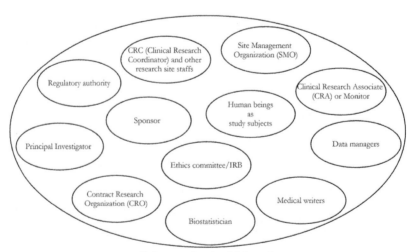

Fig: Important players in a clinical research

1.9 Reasons for Research

Research is conducted to prove or disapprove a hypothesis or to learn new facts about something. There can be many different reasons for conducting a research. Some of the common reasons are mentioned in the **Fig – Reasons to research**.

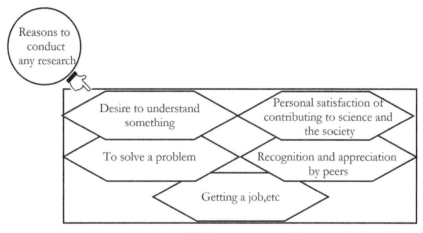

Fig: Reasons to research

1.10 Scope of Clinical Research

Clinical research is the process of using research studies intended to answer the specific health related questions. It covers study of the disease mechanisms, therapeutic interventions, epidemiology and clinical trials with an objective to understand human diseases and improving human health (refer to the **Fig – Scope of clinical research**). Thus, the clinical research involves human participants and helps to translate the basic research (done in labs) into new treatments and improvement in human health.

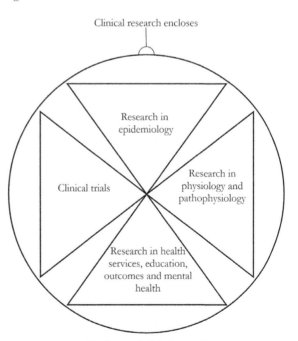

Fig: Scope of clinical research

1.11 Types of Clinical Research

There are different types of clinical research, which can be used depending upon the type of study the researcher is targeting. Some important types of clinical research are mentioned in the **Fig – Types of clinical research**.

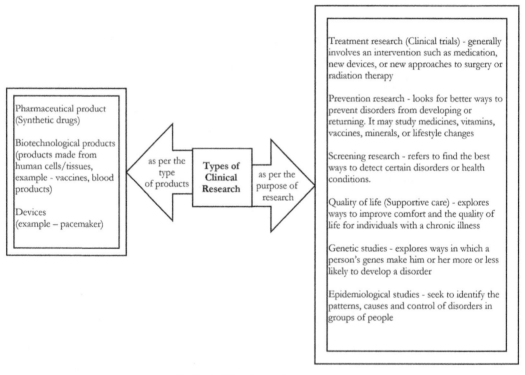

Fig: Types of clinical research

1.12 Importance of Clinical Research

Clinical research is a systematic observational and experimental biomedical study performed in human subjects in order to study drug/device/biologics/surgery/radiotherapy etc. for its safe and therapeutic use. The ultimate goal of Clinical Research is to improve the quality of life. Some of the significant contributions of clinical research in the field of medical science are listed in the **Fig – Importance of Clinical Research**.

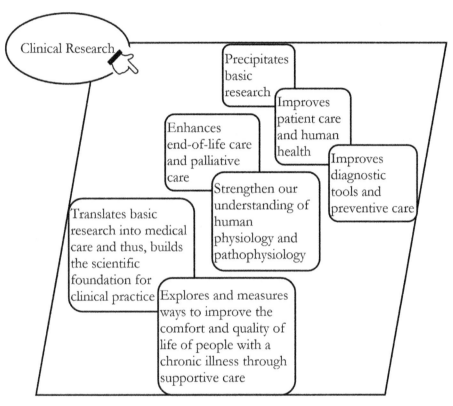

Fig - Importance of clinical research

[The end-of-life care refers to healthcare, not only for the patients in the final hours/days of their lives, but more broadly the care of all those with a terminal illness or a terminal condition that has become advanced, progressive and incurable.

Palliative care is a medical care that relieves pain/ symptoms/ stress caused by serious illnesses, thereby improving patients' quality of life. e.g. Comfort care given to a patient suffering from cancer from the time of diagnosis and throughout the duration of illness.]

1.13 Outcomes of Clinical Research

The outcome can be defined as the final result of something, or the way things end up. Outcomes of clinical research is summarized in the **Fig – Outcomes of clinical research**.

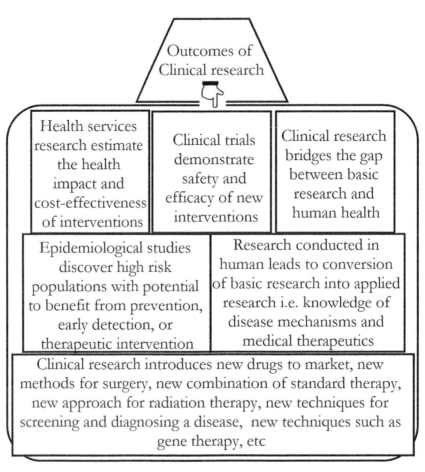

Fig: Outcomes of Clinical research

Chapter 2

HISTORY OF CLINICAL RESEARCH

2.1 Learnings from the Chapter

- *Brief history/development of human research (with respect to Clinical Research)*

2.2 Introduction

Human inquisitive nature has been the real motivation and the reason behind the development and advancement of medical science. However, the history of clinical research provides the evidence regarding the unethical practices and disregards for the well-being of human beings as study subjects. Thus, human subjects have witnessed/validated and supported the theories established in the process of advancement of medical science. There have been disasters in the past however, the mankind has bounced back with major innovations in the field of medical science. Modifications in the conduct of clinical trials and the advancement of the regulatory processes have resulted in significant improvement in patient care, safety, and clinical outcomes.

Mentioned below is the brief history of development of human research (with respect to Clinical Research)

Book of Daniel (605 B.C)

King Nebuchadnezzar believed that a diet containing meat and wine can provide a healthier life. But, Daniel and few others were not convinced with this thinking. Hence, the king did an experiment and allowed Daniel and few others to eat only vegetables and no meat and wine. On the other hand, rest of others were provided meat and wine. At the end of the 10-days experiment, the two groups were compared and Daniel and others who were on vegetarian diet were found healthier compared to others who were on meat and wine.

First Clinical Trial of Novel Therapy (1537)

Ambroise Paré, a French military surgeon, tried a combination of egg yolk, turpentine, and rose oil against the standard treatment of boiling oil for sealing soldier wounds.

First Controlled Trial (1747)

Dr. James Lind, a Scottish naval surgeon, conducted the first controlled clinical trial to treat scurvy in sailors. Lind tested six proposed remedies in twelve affected soldiers. He made six groups and then he introduced each group with different supplement in addition to their regular diet. He found that oranges and lemons were far better than the other five proposed treatments.

Placebo Effect First Demonstrated (1799)

John Haygarth conducted placebo-controlled single-blind studies in which he did a comparative study of metal rods ("Perkins tractors") with wooden rods (wooden rods were shaped and painted to look like metallic rods).

Inception of U.S. Food and Drug Administration i.e., FDA (1862)

The newly created U.S. Department of Agriculture acquired the duty of directing substance examinations of rural items (agricultural products). Afterwards, this office was known as the Food and Drug Administration (FDA).

National Institute of Health (NIH) founded (1887)

NIH is one of the largest sources of funding for medical research in the world.

U.S. Biologics Control Act Passed (1902)

The U.S. Biologics Control Act (also called the Virus-Toxin Law), allowed the federal government to control the processes used for the production of biological products. It was passed in response to the deaths of 13 children who received a diphtheria antitoxin contaminated with tetanus.

American Medical Association (AMA) started evaluating drugs (1905)

The American Medical Association (AMA) created the Council on Pharmacy and Chemistry to assess the drugs for quality and safety.

U.S. Pure Food and Drugs Act Passed (1906)

President Theodore Roosevelt signed the U.S. Pure Food and Drugs Act into law which regulated that products could not be sold outside the labeling and prohibited the interstate transport of misbranded and adultered foods, drinks, and drugs.

Double-Blinding First Used (1908)

W.H.R. Rivers did investigation of the impact of alcohol and other drugs on fatigue. He was the first to use and represent double-blinding in his study.

Invention of Human Guinea Pig Term (1913)

George Bernard Shaw invented the term "human guinea pig" to negatively compare human and animal research.

Need for Randomization First Described (1925)

R. A. Fisher, a statistician and geneticist, through his book "Statistical Methods for Research Workers" first represented the need of randomization in experimental study. He said that randomization has power to eliminate bias and provide a valid test of significance.

The Tuskegee Syphilis study (1932- 1972)

The US public Health Service conducted trials on 600 subjects to study the effects of syphilis. In this trial, neither informed consent was taken from the subjects nor they received penicillin (a proven treatment for syphilis). Because of which, many died, infected others with disease and passed congenital syphilis to their children. The study was called "Tuskegee Study of Untreated Syphilis in the Negro Male".

Sulfanilamide Disaster (1937)

Over 100 people died after the consumption of elixir sulfanilamide preparation. Elixir sulfanilamide had not been tested in humans prior to marketing. The solvent used to suspend the active ingredient was a poison. This disaster prompted passage of the U.S. Food, Drug, and Cosmetic Act (1938). It granted the U.S. Food and Drug Administration (FDA) new authority, including enforcement of the requirement that drugs must be proven safe before marketing.

Nuremberg Code Published (1947)

The Nuremberg Code was formulated in response to the atrocities of World War II. Amid World War II, prisoners were subjected to unsafe trials by German Nazi with a target to help in treating German soldiers, developing new weapons and to advance their eugenic racial ideologies. The Nuremberg Code demonstrates ten research ethics principles for research in human.

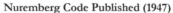

International Code of Medical Ethics Adopted (1949)

The International Code of Medical Ethics demonstrated the duties of physicians.

Birth of Institutional Review Boards (IRBs) in U.S. (1953)

The U.S. National Institutes of Health (NIH) demanded that all clinical research must be reviewed independently prior to start of study. IRB emerged as independent body to review the research including humans.

Thalidomide Disaster (1961)

Thalidomide was introduced as an effective sedative. Later, it was used for the treatment of morning sickness. The use of Thalidomide caused severe birth defects in thousands of children. This tragedy highlighted the need for rigorous testing of drugs prior to their introduction to the market. As a result of this catastrophic event, Kefauver-Harris Drug Amendments Act (1962) was implemented. This act demanded from drug manufacturers to prove the safety and effectiveness of their therapeutic product before marketing.

Declaration of Helsinki (1964)
The Declaration of Helsinki is generally regarded as the cornerstone document of human research ethics. It has been revised several times and has been codified into laws in nations around the world.

The National Research Act (1974)
According to this act, all research including human as subject should be reviewed by an Institutional Review Board in order to ensure protection of human subjects.

Society for Clinical Trials (1978)
The Society for Clinical Trials, an international professional organization, was created to develop and discuss the plan, design and analysis of clinical trials.

The Belmont Report (1979)
The Belmont Report explains three basic ethical principles i.e. Respect for persons, Beneficence and Justice to guide the research including human as subject.

International Guidelines for Biomedical Research Involving Human Subjects (1982)
The World Health Organization (WHO) and the Council for International Organizations of Medical Sciences (CIOMS) released the "International Guidelines for Biomedical Research Involving Human Subjects." The document was intended to enable countries to apply the standards of the Declaration of Helsinki and the Nuremberg Code and to provide universal guidelines which could be used globally.

The Common Rule (1991)
The Common Rule is yet another arrangement of morals which focuses on protection of human subjects. It set forth prerequisites for the Institutional Review Board's oversight of clinical trials and details protection of human subjects regarding informed consent.

MedWatch (1993)
MedWatch was launched by FDA for collection of adverse events related to medical product.

International Good Clinical Practice Guidelines (1996)
International Council for Harmonisation of Technical Requirements for Pharmaceuticals for Human Use (ICH) issued guidelines for Good Clinical Practice (GCP). ICH-GCP is a harmonized standard that "secures the rights, safety and welfare of human subjects, minimizes human exposure to investigational products, improves quality of data, accelerates marketing of new medications and decreases the cost to sponsors and to the public."

Health Insurance Portability and Accountability Act i.e. HIPAA (1996)
The demand of this act is that human participants of a research must be informed of how their protected health information will be stored and kept private during their participation in a trial.

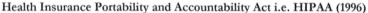

ClinicalTrials.gov Released (2000)
The U.S. National Library of Medicine (NLM), in joint effort with FDA and others, released the first version of ClinicalTrials.gov, which basically recorded clinical trials funded by the National Institutes of Health (NIH).

International Clinical Trials Registry Platform (ICTRP) Released (2007)
WHO released the first version of the International Clinical Trials Registry Platform (ICTRP) which included a search portal to access studies registered in various international registries.

European Medicine Agency (EMA) Expanded Trial Database (2013)
The European Medicines Agency (EMA) released a new version of the European Clinical Trials Database (EudraCT) to include summary results.

Chapter 3

NEED OF ETHICS, REGULATIONS AND GUIDELINES IN CLINICAL RESEARCH

3.1 Learnings from the chapter

- *Need for morals and controls in a clinical research*

- *Ethics, regulations and guidelines in detail*

- *Regulatory agencies with their responsibilities*

- *Introduction to BIMO and CIOMS*

- *Details about HIPAA and its rules*

- *ICH and GCP details*

3.2 Introduction

The study of human healthcare cannot be confined to a specific discipline as these studies cover a vast province of science. However, a perfect blend of regulations, guidelines and moral standards helps the clinical research to take place successfully. Thus, clinical research is controlled by regulations (laws) and is conducted in accordance with the prescribed guidelines and moral (ethical) considerations.

3.3 Need for morals and controls in Clinical research

The fundamental goal of clinical research is to elicit useful information and knowledge about human health and diseases by using humans as "subjects" for research. Learning from the history compels researchers to take very good care of human subjects as human, but not as an object. Use of ethical principles, guidelines and regulations ensure elimination/minimum exploitation of human subjects during research and it also takes care of respect associated with subject's welfare and rights. Thus, ethical guidelines and regulations protect human volunteers and maintain the integrity of the science.

3.4 Ethics

Ethics or moral philosophy is a branch of philosophy that involves systematizing, defending, and recommending concepts of right and wrong conduct. It is the branch of knowledge that deals with moral principles.

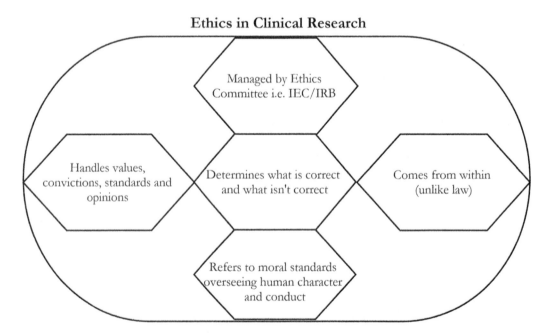

Few important codes of ethics and regulations that lead to ethical clinical research are discussed below:

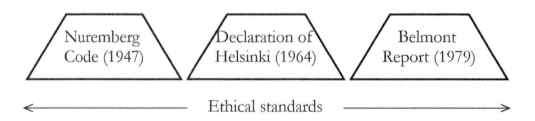

3.5 Nuremberg Code (1947)

This is a set of ethical guidelines for human experimentation which was created in light of the Nuremberg Trials led by Nazi specialists on detainees amid World War II. That was an unethical trial as researcher exposed human subjects to unsafe products. Nuremberg code was considered as the first principal international document to present guidelines on research ethics which was focused on human rights of research subjects. Principles of Nuremberg code are listed in the **Fig – Nuremberg Code – Principles**.

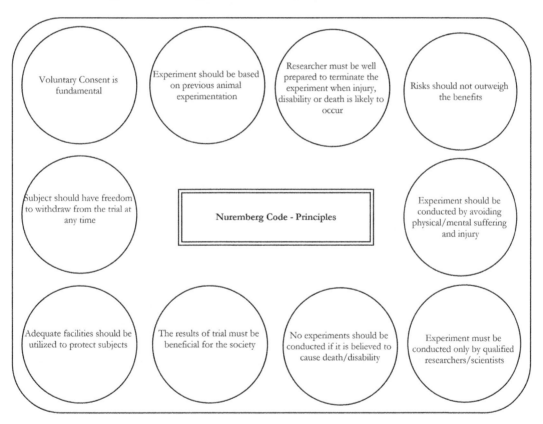

Fig: Nuremberg Code Principles

3.6 Declaration of Helsinki (1964)

This is a set of ethical guidelines regarding human experimentation developed for the medical community by the World Medical Association (WMA). It focuses on commitments of physician–investigators to look into the research subject. It underlines the difference between clinical practice and clinical research i.e., former provides direct benefit to patients but latter may or may not provide direct benefit to the human subjects. These rules have experienced numerous modifications. 12 standards of Declaration of Helsinki which direct physicians on ethical considerations identified with biomedical research are listed below:

1. Medical research including human subjects must comply with generally accepted scientific standards and it should be based on exhaustive research of the scientific literature and on sufficiently performed lab and animal experimentation.

2. The plan and execution of each step involved in an investigation (which includes human subjects), should be documented comprehensibly in a research protocol and this protocol should be submitted to a selected independent committee for thought, remark and direction.

3. Medical research involving human subjects must be conducted only by individuals who possess appropriate ethics along with the required scientific education, training and qualifications. Research on human subjects (patients or healthy volunteers) requires the supervision of a competent and appropriately qualified physician or other health care professional.

4. Medical research including human subjects should not be approved legally unless the significance of the goal is to a greater extent as compared to the inherent hazard to the subject.

5. Every medical research including the one on human subjects should be preceded by cautious evaluation of predictable risks in experiments with predictable advantages to the subject or to others. Concern for the interests of the subject should dependably beat the interests of science and society.

6. The right of the research subject to safeguard his or her integrity must always be respected. Each precautionary measure ought to be taken to regard the privacy of the subject and to limit the effect of the investigation on the subject's physical and mental integrity and on the identity of the subject.

7. Physicians should stop any experiment if the hazards are found to exceed the potential advantages. They should refrain from taking part in a research (which includes human subjects) which shows hazards involved can be unpredictable.

8. In distribution of the outcomes of his or her experiments, the researcher is obliged to protect the exactness of the outcomes. Reports of experimentation not as per the standards set down in this Declaration should not be acknowledged for publication.

9. In a medical research (which involves human beings), every potential subject must be educated enough regarding the aims, methods, foreseen advantages and potential risks of the investigation and also regarding the uneasiness it might involve. He or she should be well informed that he or she is free to withdraw from the research at any point in time. The researcher should then get the subject's freely given informed consent.

10. When obtaining informed consent for the research, the researcher should be especially careful if the subject is in dependent relationship to him or her or may consent under coercion. In such scenario, the informed consent should be obtained by a physician who isn't occupied with the research and who is totally autonomous of this official relationship.

11. In instance of legitimate inadequacy, informed consent should be obtained from the legal guardian as per national enactment. Wherever physical or mental inadequacy makes it difficult to obtain informed consent, or when the subject is a minor, an authorization from the capable relative replaces that of the subject as per national enactment. Whenever the minor child is in fact able to give a consent, the minor's consent must be obtained in addition to the consent of the minor's legal guardian.

12. The research protocol should always contain a statement of the ethical considerations included and it should demonstrate that the standards articulated in the present affirmation are complied with.

Significant changes which were found in Declaration of Helsinki but were not present in Nuremberg code are listed in the **Fig – Changes in Declaration of Helsinki as compared to Nuremberg code**. Nuremberg Code and Declaration of Helsinki became the basis for current federal regulations.

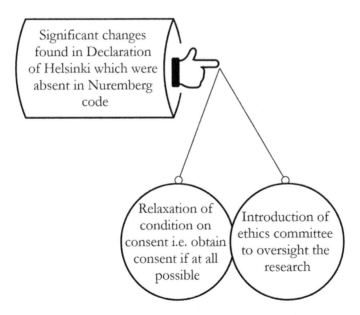

Fig: Changes in Declaration of Helsinki as compared
to Nuremberg code

3.7 Belmont Report

This report was developed in 1979 (refer to the **Fig – Belmont Report – Principles**). In response to this report, both the U.S. Department of Health and Human Services and the U.S. Food and Drug Administration revised their regulations on research studies that involve human beings.

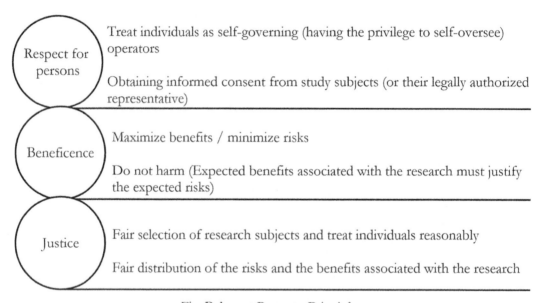

Fig: Belmont Report - Principles

3.8 Extracts of Ethical Standards

Extract of all ethical standards has been depicted in the **Fig – Extracts of Ethical Standards** which must be followed in any research.

3.9 Regulations

Regulations maintained by regulatory bodies are used to guide, manage and control the research activities in accordance with the rules led by the laws.

Effective regulation takes care of various functions in a clinical trial such as evaluation of safety and efficacy, inspection of all trial related places and activities, approval of investigational product, monitoring safety reporting, etc. Regulatory authority/agency regulates these regulations.

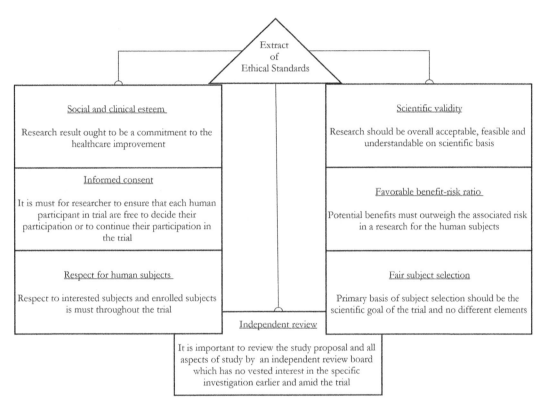

Fig: Extract of Ethical Standards

3.10 Few Regulatory Agencies

Few Regulatory Agencies (Authorities) are listed below:

Countries	Regulatory agencies
USA	FDA (Food and Drug Administration)
Europe	EMA (European Medicines Agency)
UK	MHRA (Medicines and Healthcare Products Regulatory Agency)
Canada	Health Canada
Australia	TGA (Therapeutic Goods Administration)

3.11 Important roles and responsibilities of Regulatory Agencies

Regulatory agencies play an important role throughout the lifecycle of a medicinal product. These bodies take care of the safety and well-being of the human subjects (participants in a research).

They also ensure the validity and quality of the manufactured product. Thus, these agencies look into all the aspects of a research. The roles and responsibilities of the regulatory authorities are mentioned in the **Fig – Few important roles and responsibilities of Regulatory agencies.**

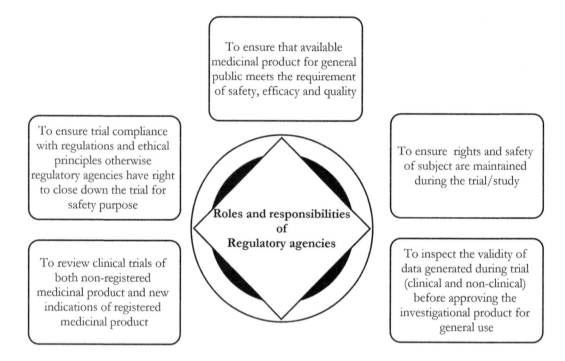

Fig: Few important roles and responsibilities of Regulatory agencies

3.12 FDA (Food and Drug Administration)

FDA (Food and Drug Administration) – An International Regulatory Agency

- The FDA is an agency within the U.S. Department of Health and Human Services.

- It oversees the manufacturing and distribution of food, pharmaceuticals, medical devices, tobacco and other consumer products and veterinary medicine.

- CDER (The Center for Drug Evaluation and Research) and CBER (The Center for Biologics Evaluation and Research) are two central laboratories which come under FDA.

- FDA Laws – CFR (Code of Federal Regulations) is divided into 50 titles and Section 21 of CFR contains regulations related to Food and Drug. 21 CFR consists of 1499 parts starting from 1
- Some important FDA regulations required for clinical research process:
  - ✓ 21 CFR Part 11 – Electronic records, Electronic signature
  - ✓ 21 CFR Part 50 – Protection of human subjects
  - ✓ 21 CFR Part 54 – Financial disclosure by clinical investigator
  - ✓ 21 CFR Part 56 – Institutional Review Board
  - ✓ 21 CFR Part 312 – Investigational new drug application
  - ✓ 21 CFR Part 314 – Application for FDA approval to market a new drug

3.13 BIMO (Bioresearch Monitoring Program)

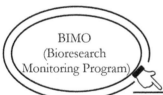

FDA program of audit/inspection

Deals with on site inspections and data audits

Designed to monitor all aspects of conduct and reporting of FDA regulated research

Oversees IRBs, investigators, sponsors, contract research organizations, monitor and others involved in a clinical trials

Assures the quality and integrity of data submitted to the agency for approval purpose of new therapeutic product

Protects the rights, safety and welfare of human subjects

3.14 HIPAA (Health Insurance Portability and Accountability Act)

HIPAA (Health Insurance Portability and Accountability Act of 1996) is a law that provides data privacy and security provisions for safeguarding medical information. It was established to improve the efficiency and effectiveness of the nation's health care system and to protect sensitive patient data. HIPAA was incepted in 1996 by Congress.

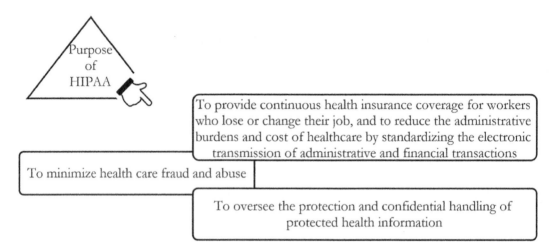

HIPAA plays an important role in clinical research studies which utilizes identifiable, personal health information (PHI). Failure to comply with HIPAA can lead to civil or even criminal sanctions against an institution or independent investigative site. HIPAA encloses following rules (refer to the **Fig – HIPAA**).

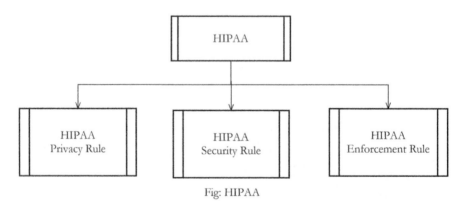

Fig: HIPAA

The Privacy rule, Security rule and Enforcement rule have been described below:

3.15 HIPAA Privacy Rule

This rule (officially known as the "Standards for Privacy of Individually Identifiable Health Information") sets up national standards to protect patient health information (PHI). It regulates the use and disclosure of Protected Health Information (PHI) held by "covered entities". Covered entities generally include employer sponsored health plans, health insurers, medical service providers that engage in certain transactions and health care clearinghouses (Entities that facilitate electronic transactions by "translating" data between health plans and providers when they use non-compatible information systems). Important features related to Privacy rule are listed in the **Fig – Features of Privacy rule**.

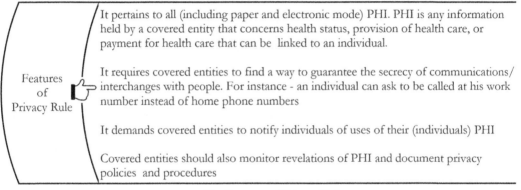

Features of Privacy Rule

It pertains to all (including paper and electronic mode) PHI. PHI is any information held by a covered entity that concerns health status, provision of health care, or payment for health care that can be linked to an individual.

It requires covered entities to find a way to guarantee the secrecy of communications/ interchanges with people. For instance - an individual can ask to be called at his work number instead of home phone numbers

It demands covered entities to notify individuals of uses of their (individuals) PHI

Covered entities should also monitor revelations of PHI and document privacy policies and procedures

Fig: Features of Privacy Rule

3.16 HIPAA Security Rule

This rule establishes national standards for securing patient data that is stored or transferred electronically. This rule complements the Privacy Rule. It deals specifically with Electronic Protected Health Information (e-PHI). It incorporates three sorts of security shields required for compliance: administrative, physical, and technical (refer to the **Fig – HIPAA Security shields**)

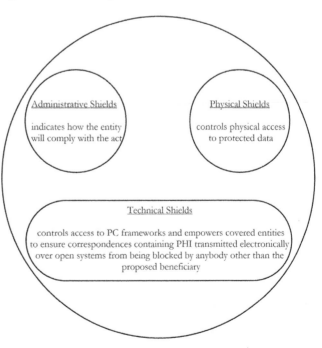

Administrative Shields

indicates how the entity will comply with the act

Physical Shields

controls physical access to protected data

Technical Shields

controls access to PC frameworks and empowers covered entities to ensure correspondences containing PHI transmitted electronically over open systems from being blocked by anybody other than the proposed beneficiary

Fig: HIPAA Security shields

3.17 HIPAA Enforcement Rule

This rule sets up guidelines for investigations concerning HIPAA compliance infringement. Some common complaints with respect to privacy against physician's practices are listed in the **Fig – Complaints with respect to privacy against physician's practices.**

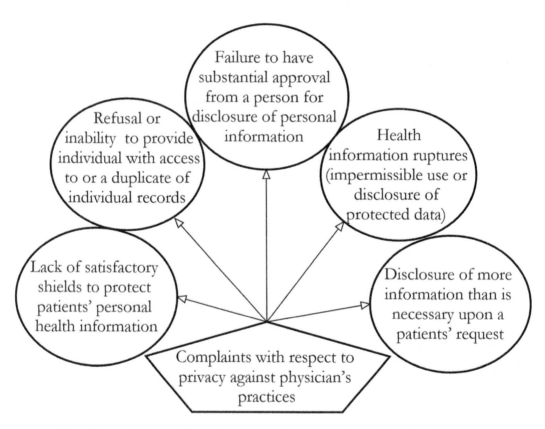

Fig: Complaints with respect to privacy against physician's practices

3.18 Guidelines

Guidelines are composed of instructions that need to be followed for standardized conduct of research. These guidelines can be made by various associations. Each country may have its own guidelines and regulations.

International Guidelines

ICH - GCP (International Council for Harmonisation - Good Clinical Practice)

CIOMS (Council for International Organizations of Medical Sciences) Guidelines
(created jointly by WHO and UNESCO)

3.19 GCP (Good Clinical Practice)

GCP is a set of ethical and scientific quality standard guidelines for biomedical studies which encompasses the design, conduct, performance, monitoring, recording, analysis, reporting and documentation of the studies involving human subjects.

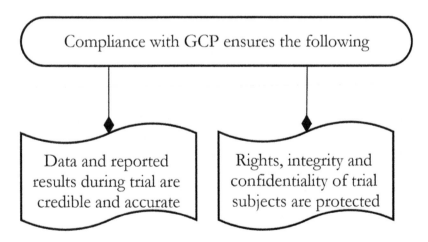

Compliance with GCP ensures the following

Data and reported results during trial are credible and accurate

Rights, integrity and confidentiality of trial subjects are protected

3.20 Role of GCPs in Clinical Research

Clinical trial must be conducted in accordance with GCP standards. Clinical studies which are compliant with GCP standards ensures that the rights, safety and well-being of study subjects are protected and the studies are consistent with the ethical principles. It also ensures the production of valid and credible clinical data. Important roles of GCPs in a clinical research are depicted in the **Fig – GCP (Good Clinical Practice).**

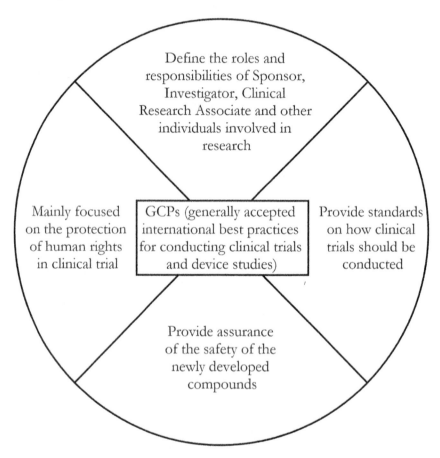

Fig: GCP (Good Clinical Practice)

3.21 ICH (International Council for Harmonisation)

ICH (International Council for Harmonisation of Technical Requirements for Pharmaceuticals for Human Use)

Earlier, "International Council for Harmonization" was called "International Conference on Harmonization". The new form of ICH (International Council for Harmonization) was officially established on October 23, 2015. The reformation of ICH has a more stable operating structure through the establishment of an ICH association (a legal entity under Swiss law).

ICH was established in April 1990, in Brussels. ICH brought together the regulatory authorities and pharmaceutical industry of Europe, Japan and the US to discuss scientific and technical aspects of drug registration. The four categories of ICH guidelines are mentioned in the **Fig – Categories of ICH guidelines.**

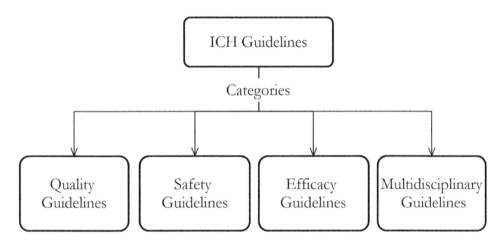

Fig: Categories of ICH Guidelines

3.22 Objectives of ICH

The ultimate objective of ICH is harmonization for better health. Harmonization would result into an efficient use of human, animal and material resources. It helps to maintain the safeguards on quality, safety, efficacy and regulatory obligations to protect public health. Some of the important objectives are listed in the **Fig – Objectives of ICH.**

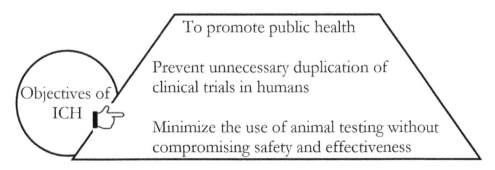

Fig: Objectives of ICH

3.23 Goal of ICH

ICH provides a central stage for the global pharmaceutical regulatory harmonization. It brings together all the key regulatory authorities and industry stakeholders in a transparent manner. Major goals of ICH are listed in the **Fig – Goals of ICH**.

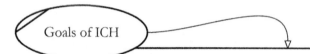

Promote international harmonization by bringing together representatives from the three ICH regions (EU, Japan and USA) to discuss and establish common guidelines

Promote mutual understanding regarding regional initiatives to maintain harmonization related to ICH guidelines regionally and globally and to strengthen the capacity of drug regulatory authorities and industry to utilize them

Provide information on request by any company/country regarding guidelines/ activities of ICH

Fig: Goals of ICH

3.24 The Principles of ICH – GCP

- Clinical trials should be conducted as per the ethical principles that have their origin in the Declaration of Helsinki, and that are consistent with GCP and the applicable regulatory requirement(s).

- Before a trial is initiated, foreseeable risks and inconveniences should be weighed against the anticipated benefit for the individual trial subject and society. A trial should be initiated and continued only if the anticipated benefits justify the risks.

- The rights, safety, and well-being of the trial subjects are the most imperative considerations and should beat the interests of science and society.

- The available nonclinical and clinical information on an investigational product should be adequate to support the proposed clinical trial.

- Clinical trials should be logically stable (scientifically sound), and described in a clear, detailed protocol.

- A trial should be conducted in compliance with the protocol that has received prior institutional review board (IRB)/independent ethics committee (IEC) approval.

- The restorative care given to, and therapeutic choices made for the benefit of subjects, should dependably be the duty of a qualified doctor or, when fitting, of a qualified dental specialist.

- Each individual involved in conducting a trial should be qualified by education, training, and experience to perform his or her respective task(s).

- Freely given informed consent should be obtained from every subject preceding clinical trial participation.

- All clinical trial information should be recorded, handled, and stored in a way that permits its precise reporting, interpretation and verification.

- The confidentiality of records that could identify subjects should be protected, respecting the privacy and confidentiality rules in accordance with the applicable regulatory requirement(s).

- Investigational products should be manufactured, handled, and stored in accordance with applicable good manufacturing practice (GMP). They should be used in accordance with the approved protocol.

- Systems with procedures that guarantee the quality of every aspect of the trial should be implemented.

3.25 CIOMS (Council for International Organizations of Medical Sciences)

The Council for International Organizations of Medical Sciences (CIOMS) is an international, non-governmental, non-profit organization established jointly by WHO and UNESCO in 1949. The prime objective of CIOMS is to improve public health through guidance on health research including ethics, medical product development and safety.

Development of CIOMS

CIOMS are international guidelines which play imperative role in the field of medical research. The CIOMS guidelines directs different aspects related to research such as informed consent, standards for external review, recruitment of participants, etc. These guidelines are general instructions and principles of ethical biomedical research. Development of CIOMS is depicted in the **Fig – Development of CIOMS.**

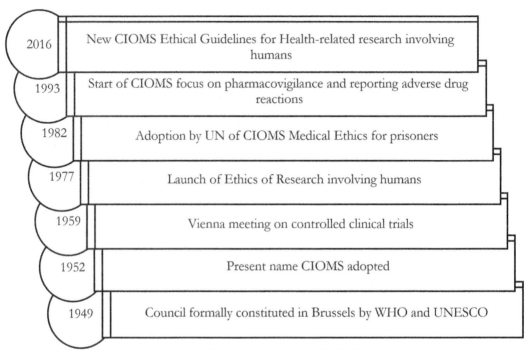

Fig: Development of CIOMS

Chapter 4

CLINICAL RESEARCH – VARIOUS DESIGNS

4.1 Learnings from the chapter

- *Definition of research design*

- *Details about qualitative and quantitative research*

- *Different types of research design (i.e., descriptive study, observational study, study/review of other research and experimental study)*

- *Selection of research design and importance of appropriate research design*

4.2 Introduction

A research design is the framework of a research study. It explains how an investigation will take place. It provides a logical sequence of the investigation which is needed to be followed to achieve the desired outcome. A research design presents a detailed outline with key features of the work to be undertaken, methods of data collection and analysis to be employed. It shows how the research strategy will address the specific aims and objectives of the study.

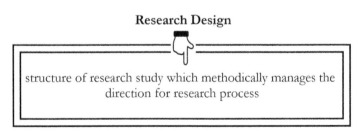

Research Design

structure of research study which methodically manages the direction for research process

With the help of a research design, the researcher can ensure that the proposed investigation is feasible within the research environment and the timeframe defined for the research. It also furnishes other players of the research with the understanding of the investigation plan.

4.3 Classification of clinical studies (research)

All clinical studies (researches) can be classified into intervention studies (experimental studies) and non-intervention studies (observational studies) [refer to the **Fig – Clinical studies (research)**].

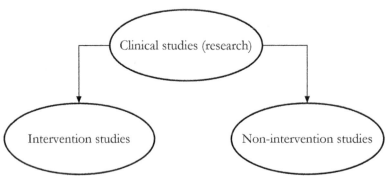

Fig: Clinical studies (research)

However, there are various research designs which fall under these two [Non-intervention/ Observational and Intervention /Experimental studies] categories. Selecting the appropriate design out of multiple choices of the research design can be a challenging task because a design can impact the results and findings of a study. There are many factors which must be taken into consideration such as the research question, ethics, budget, time, etc. while selecting a research design.

4.4 Qualitative research and Quantitative research

Regardless of the research topic, researchers have just two sorts of research approaches to browse i.e. qualitative research and quantitative research. Each of these have their own particular qualities and shortcomings (refer to the **Fig – Approaches to research**).

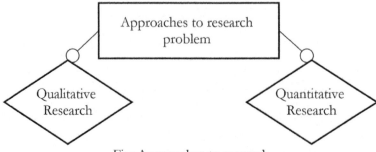

Fig: Approaches to research

Features of Qualitative and Quantitative research

Qualitative research	Quantitative research
Exploratory in nature - provides a complete, detailed description of the research topic	Confirmatory/conclusive in nature - focuses more on checking and arranging highlights and building measurable models and figures to clarify what is observed
Perfect for initial phases of research projects	Perfect for later phases of research projects
Utilized when we do not know what to expect, how to characterize the issue or how to build up a way to deal with the issue	Used to evaluate an issue and to see how predominant it is by searching for projectable outcomes to a bigger populace
More subjective [depicts an issue or condition from the perspective of those encountering it]	More objective [provides observed effects (interpreted by researchers) of a program on an issue or condition]
Principally inductive process used to figure theories or hypothesis with the information	Principally deductive process used to test the pre-indicated hypothesis and theory with the information
Content based i.e., information can be observed yet can't be measured hence, statistical tests cannot be used	Number based i.e., information can be measured using statistical tests
Unstructured or semi-organized methods utilized e.g. individual depth interviews or group discussions, reviews of documents	Structured methods utilized e.g. surveys, structured interviews & observations, reviews of records or archives for numeric information
Generally, relies upon aptitude and thoroughness of the researcher	Generally, relies upon the measurement device or instrument utilized
Less probability of getting generalized	Higher probability of getting generalized
Builds up an underlying understanding	Prescribes a final strategy

If a researcher plans to discover an answer to a research question through numerical proof, then the use of the Quantitative Research is advisable. However, an investigation which intends to clarify further on why this specific occasion happened, or why this specific phenomenon has occurred, for such a research the use of Qualitative Research is advisable (refer to the **Fig – Quantitative research & Qualitative research**).

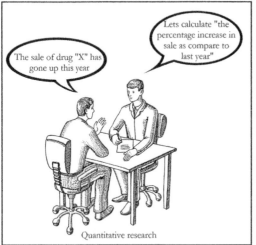 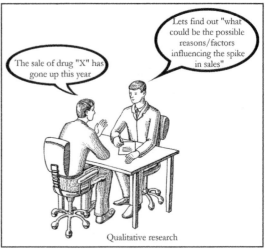

Fig: Quantitative research & Qualitative research

In few investigations, utilization of both Quantitative and Qualitative Research is required. For example, in case of a study which intends to look at what the predominant human conduct is towards a specific occasion and at the same time it intends to analyse why this situation exists, for such a situation, it is advisable to make use of both techniques.

4.5 Different Research Design

There are number of research designs which can be used in a clinical research, all having their own advantages and disadvantages. Some major designs (refer to the **Fig – Types of research designs**) are discussed in this chapter.

Fig: Types of research designs

4.6 Descriptive Study

Descriptive study describes some of the functions or characteristics of a phenomenon without changing the environment (i.e., nothing is manipulated). The purpose of descriptive study is to gather information concerning the current status of the phenomena in order to describe "what exists" with respect to variables/conditions in a situation. Important features of Descriptive study are mentioned in the **Fig – Features of Descriptive study.**

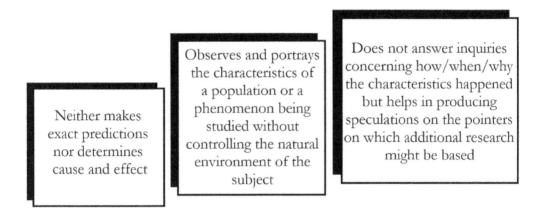

Fig:Features of Descriptive study

Types of Descriptive study

The various types of descriptive study i.e., naturalistic observation, laboratory observation, case studies, survey (refer to the **Fig – Types of Descriptive Study**) have been discussed below:

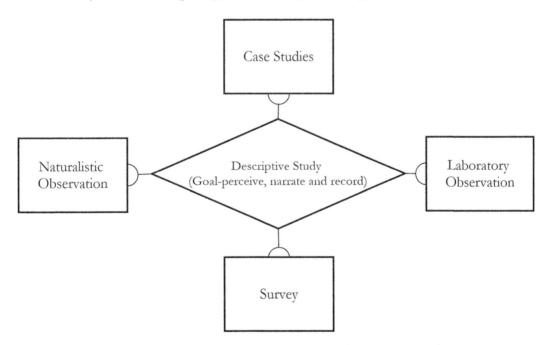

Fig: Types of Descriptive Study

4.7 Naturalistic Observation

Subject is observed by researcher in its common setting with no manipulation, hence, there is no interference with the subject's behaviour. Study happens in real-life setting so reasonable outcomes can be expected. The purpose of naturalistic observation is to observe the study subjects in a natural environment.

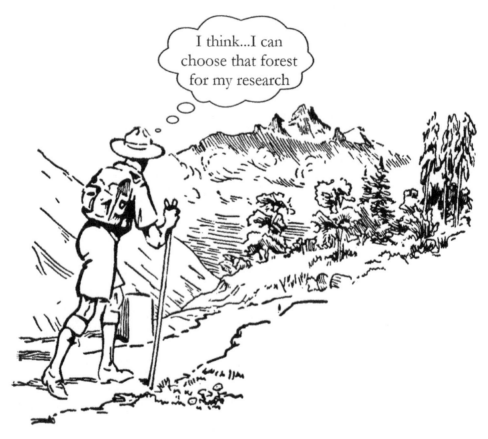

Example of naturalistic observation - Dian Fossey's study of the mountain gorilla; she did extensive study of the mountain gorillas for nearly 20 years and she explained that gorillas are kind and social beings having curiosity and affection.

4.8 Laboratory Observation

Subject is observed in a laboratory and researcher can concentrate intently on subject's characteristics without any interference. It allows more control than naturalistic observation however confines reality. This kind of study can produce unnatural results as it occurs in artificial setting. The purpose of laboratory observation is to observe the study subjects in a controlled environment.

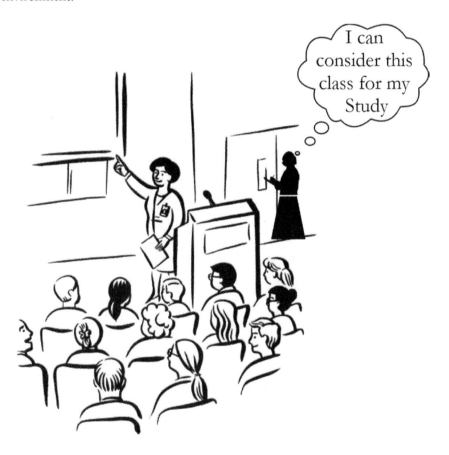

Laboratory observation of behaviour of students during class hour in a classroom of a college (here classroom is the laboratory and students are study subjects)

Example- The Marshmallow Test; Walter Mischel and his team did a laboratory observation with pre-school kids to find out whether kids could wait before eating a single marshmallow long enough to earn two marshmallows. In this experiment, the preschool kids were called to a room by an instructor. They were told that the instructor is going to leave the room and will be back in sometime. The instructor informed the children that if they wanted to have the marshmallows right now, they may have it, however, they can have two marshmallows if they opt to have marshmallows when the instructor comes back. Then, the instructor leaves the room and the researchers observe the kids behind a one-way mirror.

4.9 Case Study

An individual or group of individuals will be investigated in-depth to understand a specific case. Hence, this study cannot be generalized to a bigger populace and is useful to limit an extremely wide field of research into one effectively researchable topic and also to study rare phenomena.

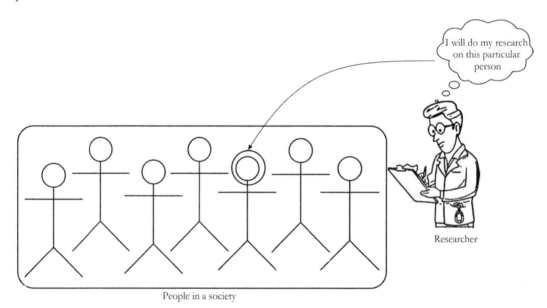

People in a society

This study gathers data by investigating portrayal of individual's encounters and contemplations with respect to the topic being examined. It does not prove or disapprove anything but it incorporates innovativeness, provides different viewpoints and delivers considerably detailed results. Case study does not provide answer to an inquiry totally however it provides a few signs and permits advance elaboration and theory creation regarding a particular topic.

Example – Koluchova (1976) reported the consequences of childhood deprivation on later emotional and cognitive development in a set of twin boys; he studied the identical twin boys who had been isolated and cruelly treated for 5 ½ years by their stepmother. By the time they were found by a child care agency, the twins were dwarfed in stature, suffered from rickets, lacked speech and scared of people and normal objects.

4.10 Survey

Survey comprises of interviews, questionnaires or a blend of the two. In survey, participants answer the questions asked to them through interviews or questionnaires. Their responses will later be portrayed by researchers. Hence, questions should be framed appropriately to make study results reliable and valid. Survey may work for factual information about individuals or may collect opinion of survey takers.

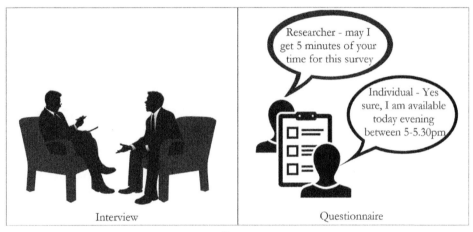

Survey

4.11 Observation Study

An observational study draws inferences from a sample to a population where the independent variable is not under the control of the researcher because of ethical concerns or logistical constraints. Important features of Observation Study are mentioned in the **Fig – Features of Observation Study.**

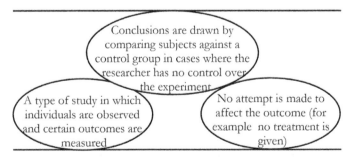

Fig: Features of Observation Study

Types of observation study

Different types of observational study i.e., cohort studies, case-control studies, cross-sectional studies (refer to the **Fig – Types of Observation study**) have been discussed below:

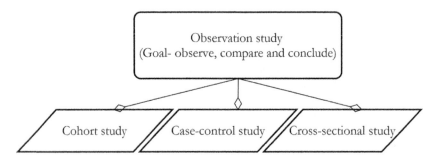

Fig: Types of observation Study

4.12 Cohort study

A cohort study is a study that observes a particular group with a certain trait over a period of time. Thus, a defined group of patients (having some specific characteristics "A") is observed for a defined period of time simultaneously with another group (characterized with absence of characteristic "A") to read the outcome. This study is prospective in nature.

   Example - A study is conducted to compare the outcomes of one group which is exposed to smoking habit (smokers) with the outcomes of another group which is not exposed to smoking habit (non-smokers). Both the groups are simply observed (without any interference/intervention) over a period of time and the outcomes are compared. (refer to the **Fig – Cohort Studies**).

4.13 Case control study

A study that compares patients who have a disease or outcome of interest (cases) with patients who do not have the disease or outcome (controls), and it looks back retrospectively to compare frequency of the exposure to a risk factor for each group to estimate the relationship between the risk factor and the disease. Case control studies are also known as "retrospective studies" and "case-referent studies."

Example - Few cancer patients and non- cancer patients are selected and the history of both groups are studied to compare the frequency of exposure to risk factors for each group in order to estimate the relationship between the risk factor and the disease (refer to the **Fig- Case Control Studies**).

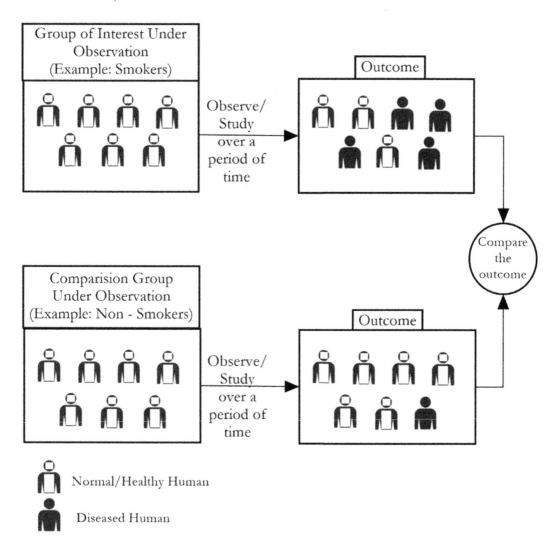

Fig: Cohort Studies

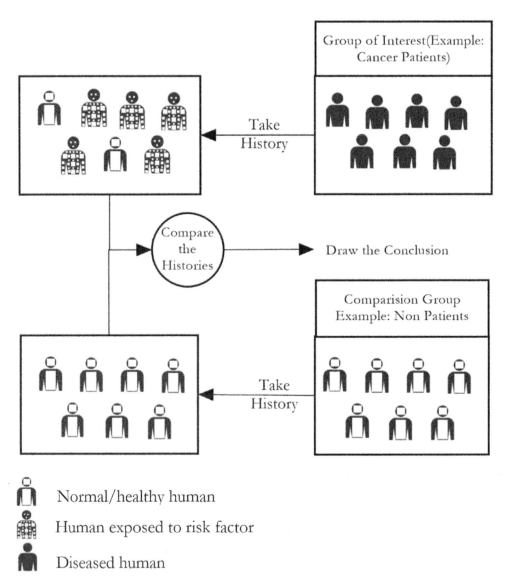

Fig: Case-control studies

4.14 Cross-sectional study

Cross-sectional study is a type of observational study that analyses the data collected from a population, or a representative subset, at a specific point in time. This study takes a snapshot of a population at a certain time, allowing the conclusions about the phenomena across a wide population to be drawn. Cross-sectional study can compare different population groups at a single point in time and it also allows the comparisons of many different variables at the same time.

Example - Measure cholesterol levels in daily walkers across two age groups, over 45 and under 45, and compare these to cholesterol levels among non-walkers across the same age groups. However, the past or future cholesterol levels are not considered in the study population, only the cholesterol levels at one point in time (present) are considered (refer to the **Fig – Cross-sectional study**).

The cross-sectional study is the study for a single point of time (does not consider what happens before and after the study), it does not depict a definite information about cause-effect relationships. Therefore, in the above example, it would be difficult to estimate that daily walking helped to reduce cholesterol levels that were high previously.

In short, the cross-sectional study is done to study prevalence (proportion of a specific population having a particular disease).

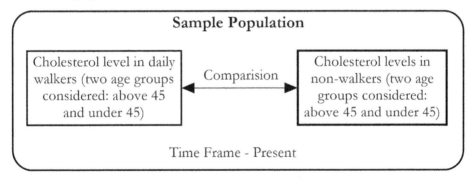

Fig: Cross sectional study

4.15 Reviewing Other Research

Research is a systematic way to find answers to a question. It can be done through conducting a research or through review of other researches which have already been done i.e. through literature review, systematic review or meta-analysis of other researches.

Types of reviewing other research

Different kinds of reviewing of other research i.e., Literature Review, Systematic Review, Meta-analysis (refer to the **Fig – Kinds of reviewing other research**) have been described below:

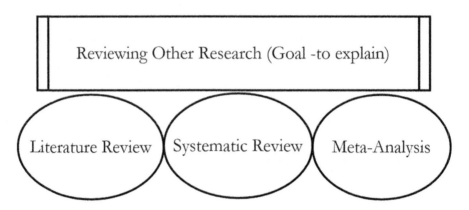

Fig: Kinds of reviewing other research

4.16 Literature Review

• Literature review is a search and evaluation of major writings and other sources (scholarly journal articles, books, government reports, Web sites, etc.) on a selected topic.

• It might give a new interpretation of old material or combine new with old interpretations.

• It ensures that researcher is familiar with the research topic before starting the research.

• It summarizes and synthesizes the information and ideas of others without adding new contributions.

4.17 Systematic Review

• Systematic review is a type of literature review that follows systematic steps to collect and critically analyze multiple research studies or papers.

• It is more comprehensive and systematic way of evaluation of previous studies compared to standard literature review.

• It is considered more reliable and accurate than individual studies but time-consuming process.

4.18 Meta – Analysis

• Meta-analysis refers to the analysis of analyses and a subset of systematic review.

- It is a statistical procedure for combining data from multiple studies to obtain an overall effectiveness of interventions, the relative impact of independent variables and the strength of relationship between variables.

- When the treatment effect (or effect size) is consistent from one study to the next, meta-analysis can be used to identify this common effect.

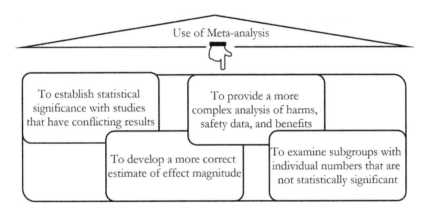

4.19 Experimental Study

Experimental study is a systematic and scientific approach to research in which the researcher manipulates one or more variables, controls and measures any change in other variables. Experimental study can be classified as true experimental study and semi experimental study (refer to the **Fig – Types of Experimental study**).

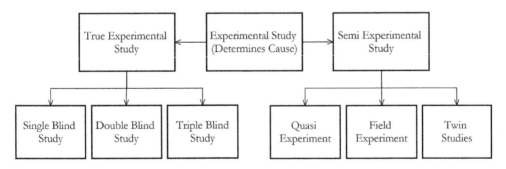

Fig: Types of Experimental Study

The different types of experimental study i.e., true experimental study and semi experimental study have been described below:

4.20 True Experimental Study

- True experimental study (Clinical trial) is regarded as the most accurate form of experimental research which involves manipulation of an independent variable to assess the effect upon dependent variables. It involves random selection of subjects and random assignment of subjects to control and experimental groups (refer to the **Fig – True Experiment**).

- Important features of a true experiment are manipulation of variable, use of control and use of randomization.

- True experimental study can be single blind study, double blind study or triple blind study (refer to the **Fig – Single, Double and Triple Blind Study**).

4.21 Single blind, Double blind and Triple blind study

Apart from the blind studies, sometimes open label studies can also be considered where every player of the trial will be aware of the treatment assignment.

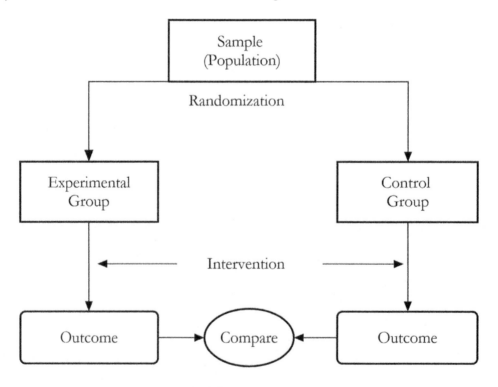

Fig: True Experiment

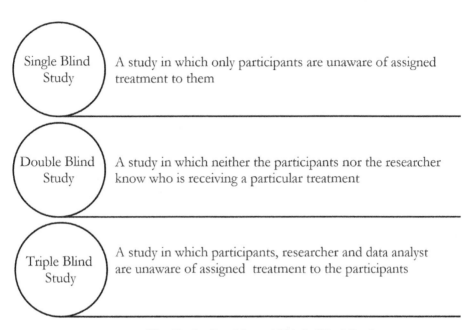

Fig: Single, Double and Triple Blind Study

4.22 Semi-experimental study

It includes Quasi experiment, Field experiment and Twin study. The types of semi experimental study have been described below:

4.23 Quasi- Experiment

This experiment involves an intervention i.e., manipulation of independent variable to study the effect on the dependent variable (like true experiment) but this experiment "lacks randomization" (unlike true experiment). This means that quasi-experiment involves assignment of study subjects to control and experimental group without use of randomization. (refer to the **Fig – True Experiment Vs Quasi Experiment**).

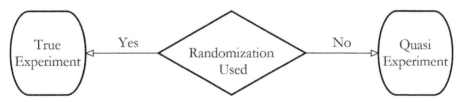

Fig: True Experiment Vs. Quasi Experiment

4.24 Types of Quasi - Experiment

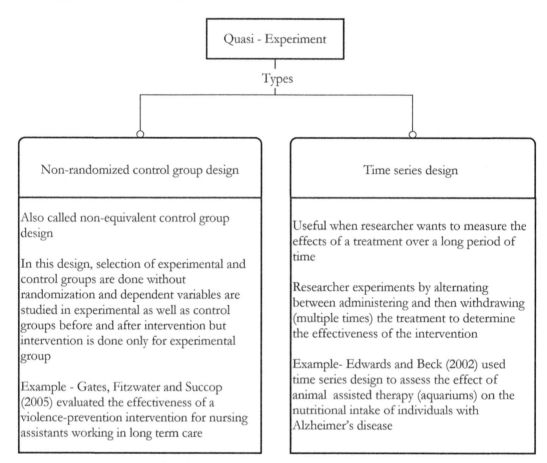

Fig: Types of Quasi - Experiment

4.25 Field Experiment

- A field experiment applies the scientific method to experimentally examine an intervention in the real world rather than in the laboratory.

- The researchers do manipulation in the independent variable to study the impact on dependent variable, but this experiment takes place in a real-life environment outside the laboratory. Thus, the researchers cannot really control the extraneous variables (unlike lab experiments) and hence this experiment is called Field experiment.

- Example - Hofling (1966) did a study of obedience by carrying out field studies on nurses who were unaware that they were involved in an experiment. The aim of this experiment was to see if the nurses would do something told by their higher authorities even if it meant their professional standards were being compromised. Hofling concluded from the experiment that people are very unwilling to question supposed 'authority', even when they have the reason and ability to do so.

4.26 Twin Study

- This study evaluates the effect of environment and genetics on human behaviour. It also studies the subsequent development by comparing the traits of identical and fraternal twins (refer to the **Fig – Identical twins and Fraternal twins**) and then comparing the twins of both kinds who have been raised together or apart. Identical twins share all of their genes, while fraternal twins share only about half (50 percent) of their genes.

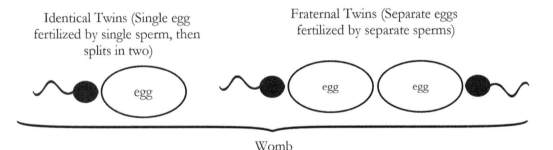

Fig: Identical twins and Fraternal twins

- Example - Mack and colleagues discovered the concordance of Hodgkin's disease in twins over a period of years. It was discovered when first twin was detected with cancer. They wanted to study if there is any difference in the frequency of occurrence of the cancer in the second twin in case of monozygotic twins and dizygotic twins. They followed up sets of twins (both monozygotic i.e., identical twins and dizygotic i.e., non-identical twins) in which one twin had Hodgkin's disease. They found that second twin of a monozygotic twins are at higher risk to develop cancer but second twin of dizygotic twins did not have any measurable increased risk to developed cancer. This study concluded that genetic factors plays an important role in the development of this type of cancer.

4.27 Pilot study

Pilot Study

Pilot Study is small scale test study which need to be done before conducting any full-scale study. The goal of Pilot study is to assure that the chosen research design will work. It also evaluates feasibility, time, cost, adverse events and effect size (statistical variability). Thus, it provides a way for required adjustments before finalizing the research design.

4.28 Selection of Research Design

Once the research question is finalized, the research design needs to be chosen with the help of research personnel and other important contributors. As discussed above, clinical research can be conducted through various designs.

It is important to give sufficient time for careful and thorough planning of any investigation so that the objectives of the study can be achieved completely and correctly. Selection of an appropriate research design for a particular trial is one of the important aspect in a trial as it forms the foundation of quality clinical research.

4.29 Importance of choosing an appropriate research design

A well-designed trial makes the analysis process easier. The design of a trial is much more important than the analysis of clinical data because a poorly analysed data can be corrected by re-analysing or with some modifications to reach the meaningful results, but in case of poorly designed trial, it is difficult to recover. Furthermore, the design of the trial selects the analysis method for that particular trial. Hence, selection of appropriate study design can impact the research positively as whole (refer to the **Fig – Importance of appropriate research design**).

4.30 Factors to be considered for deciding the Research Design

Selection of research design depends on various factors. Some of those factors are mentioned in the **Fig – Factors to be considered for deciding the research design.**

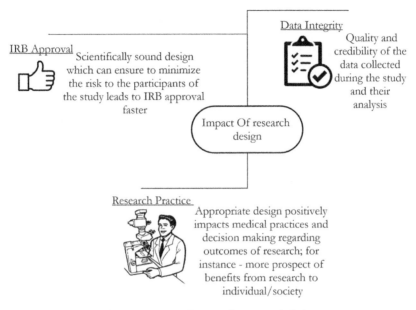

Fig: Importance of appropriate research design

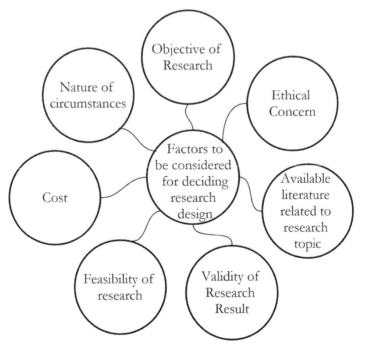

Fig: Factors to be considered for deciding the research design

4.31 Considerations to choose an appropriate design

To choose an appropriate design for a successful research completion, the researcher must consider all the important aspects of an experiment. Some of those aspects are noted below in the **Fig – Considerations to choose an appropriate research design**.

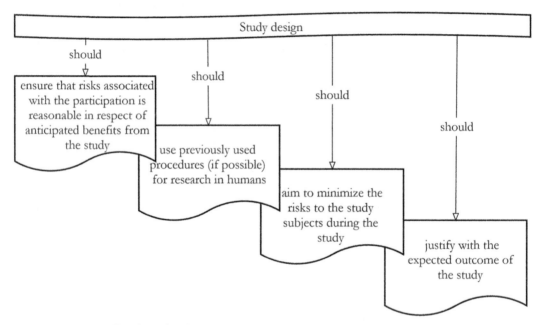

Fig: Considerations to choose an appropriate research design

4.32 How to choose an appropriate study design

While selecting a research/study design, the researcher needs to find answers to certain questions such as requirement of intervention (e.g., an experimental drug) in a study or requirement of any type of comparison for analysis process.

Depending upon the requirements of a study, the appropriate designs can be chosen to proceed in the research process. The below diagram (**Fig – Generic selection process of research design**) depicts the selection process of research design which is generic in nature.

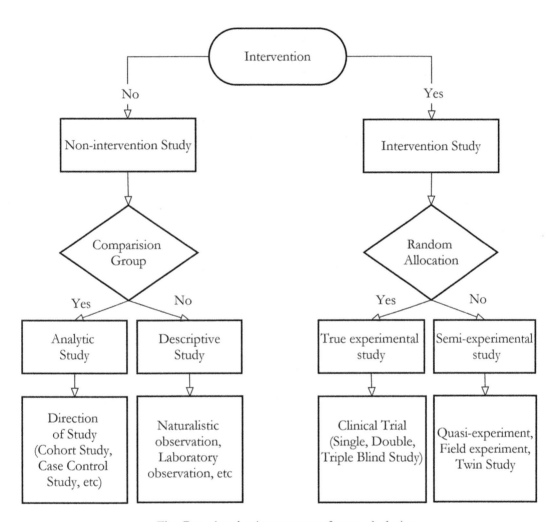

Fig: Generic selection process of research design

Chapter 5

CLINICAL TRIAL – OVERVIEW

5.1 Learnings from the chapter

- *Introduction to Clinical trial and details about its different phases and different types*

- *Concept of Randomized Controlled Trial (RCT) and its importance*

- *Commonly used designs (Parallel, Cross-over and Factorial design) in RCT*

- *Clinical trial process overview (with few aspects discussed in detail such as formulation of research question, formulation of objectives and hypothesis, etc.)*

5.2 Introduction

Clinical trial (true experiment) is a kind of clinical research which aims at originating new ways of treatments and thus contributes in improvement of health and quality of life. Clinical trial is one of the type of intervention trial (study) which involves human beings as study subjects (healthy volunteers or patients) and tests the safety and efficacy of a new treatment (i.e., a medicine, a medical device, a surgical procedure or a test for diagnosing an illness).

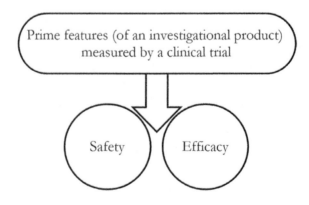

5.3 Intervention Trials

Intervention trials are clinical studies which are believed to provide strongest evidence for a proposed hypothesis. Because of ethical constraints (due to the involvement of humans as study subjects), these trials can be conducted only when there is a strong base for potential benefit to humans. The main feature of these studies is that investigator can control the intervention and allocation of study subjects (unlike non-intervention trial). The purpose of an interventional trial is to evaluate one or more new treatments for a disease/condition and thus to improve the condition of an individual or a group of individuals.

It is mandatory to collect enough data about pre-clinical studies (studies involving animals) prior to the introduction of investigational drug into human thereby ensuring that it is safe to experiment new entity into human.

5.4 Types of Clinical Trial

Clinical trials must be conducted in order to determine the benefits and risks associated with a new medicinal product. A clinical trial can compare whether a new treatment is better than existing alternatives or not. 'Better' in this context does not necessarily mean 'with a better efficacy' but it may also indicate side effects (adverse drug reactions), better handling, less burden, etc. Thus, a clinical trial can be designed with an aim to discover the superiority, equivalence or non-inferiority of an investigational product with an existing treatment. Hence, clinical trials can be of following types (refer to the **Fig – Types of clinical trial**) depending upon the objective of the research (trial).

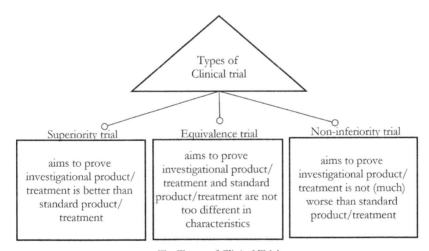

Fig: Types of Clinical Trial

5.5 Clinical trial phases

The clinical trials test the potential treatments (drug, device or biologics like vaccines) in human volunteers or patients to see whether they should be further investigated or approved for wider use in the general population or not. Clinical trials follow a typical series from small-scale studies to large scale studies (refer to the **Fig – Phases of clinical trial**).

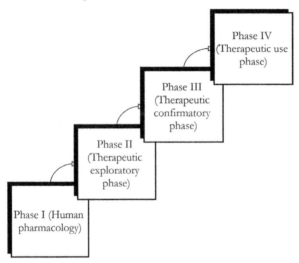

Fig: Phases of clinical trial

Clinical trials are divided into different stages which are known as "phases". These phases are built on one another. Each phase is designed to answer certain questions. The earliest phase of the trial may determine the safety profile and the side effects associated with the investigational product. The later phase of the trial may determine whether a new treatment is better than existing one or not.

Sometimes, phases of the trial are executed together (at the same time) i.e. some of the trials cover just one phase while some trials cover more than one phase. For instance, one trial can comprise both phase I and phase II where phase I tries to demonstrate the highest safe dose of an investigational product and phase II tries to find out how well the recommended dose will work.

The movement from one phase to the next phase depends on the outcome of the previous phase. There could be chances of taking a decision to stop or terminate the trial in any of the phases and this could be due to different reasons such as appearance of adverse reaction, financial issues, etc. Sometimes, a remarkable performance of candidate drug can be the reason to stop the trial in order to make available the new drug to the general public at the earliest. All four phases of a clinical trial are listed below with their important features.

5.6 Phase I (Human pharmacology)

In Phase I trial, the candidate drug is tested in human beings for the first time. The main objective of this phase is to discover the safety profile of the investigational drug in human body. The important features of Phase I are listed in the **Fig – Features of Phase I (Human pharmacology)**.

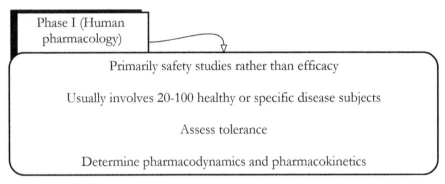

Fig: Features of Phase I (Human pharmacology)

5.7 Phase II (Therapeutic exploratory phase)

In Phase II trial, the efficacy of candidate drug will be explored in patients with target disease. Thus, the objective of this phase is to demonstrate the efficacy of the candidate drug in human body. The important features of Phase II are depicted in the **Fig – Features of Phase II (Therapeutic exploratory phase).**

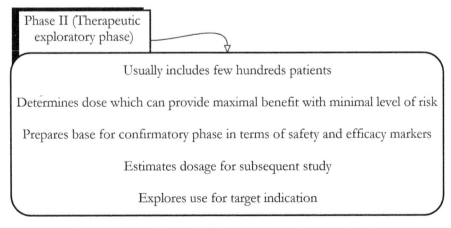

Fig: Features of Phase II (Therapeutic exploratory phase)

5.8 Phase III (Therapeutic confirmatory phase)

In phase III trial, candidate drug will be studied in large group of patients to establish safety and efficacy of the new compound. This phase produces statistically significant data about safety, efficacy, rare side effects. It also determines the relationship between the benefits and risks associated with the new compound. This phase can include comparative studies (against placebo/standard treatments) to establish the drug efficacy. Phase III trials are both the longest and the costliest trials. The important features of Phase III are mentioned in the **Fig – Features of Phase III (Therapeutic confirmatory phase)**.

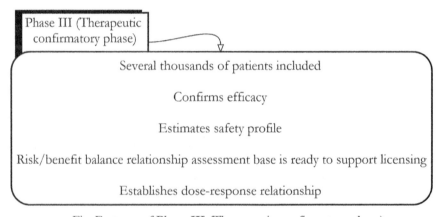

Fig: Features of Phase III (Therapeutic confirmatory phase)

Upon the completion of phase III clinical trials with successful results (i.e., the safety and efficacy of investigational drug is determined), the manufacturing company files a New Drug Application (NDA) with the FDA, with a request to approve the new drug to the market. FDA reviews all the information provided by the drug developer and if it finds everything satisfactory, it approves the company for marketing the drug.

Scaling - up for manufacturing - During clinical trial, the drugs are manufactured in small quantities while for launching the drug in the market, large scale production of the new drug is required and this is tough task for the manufacturing company. Hence, careful planning along with proper coordination is essential to run this operation smoothly.

5.9 Phase IV (Therapeutic use phase)

Post approval, even after the FDA approval is obtained and the drug has been launched in the market, the research on a new medicine continues. It is the responsibility of manufacturer and even the regulatory requirement mandates to collect information on the newly launched drug and also to monitor the adverse effects (associated with the new product) in the larger population [refer to the **Fig – Features of Phase IV (Therapeutic use phase)**].

Sometimes, the FDA needs additional studies on the already approved drug. These studies are known as Phase IV trials. These trials can be set up to evaluate the long-term safety of the new medicine. Even the manufacturer can also show interest in conducting such studies to assess the drug's potential benefits in other disease areas or for special populations (e.g., children, the elderly) or for some other reasons.

Phase IV (Therapeutic use phase)

Long term study which occurs after the marketing authorization is granted for the new medicinal product and the new product is placed onto the market

Provides additional information for safety and efficacy profile

Redefines risk/benefit relationship understanding in general/special population and special environment

Refines dosing recommendation

Identifies rare ADR and particular children's studies

Facilitates marketing research or pharmacoeconomic studies in relation to competitor drugs to assist sales

Investigates a specific adverse event or unexpected signal occurring during post-marketing

Fig: Features of Phase IV (Therapeutic use phase)

5.10 Clinical Trial – Process overview

Clinical trials are organized by researchers to answer the specific questions related to a medical product/condition. Trial typically begins with the development of a clinical protocol, which outlines how the trial will be conducted, including the objectives, design, methodology and organization. Whole clinical trial process can be divided into five parts (Refer to the **Fig – Clinical trial – Process overview**). Each part consists of various tasks which needs to be completed efficiently in order to achieve the research goals.

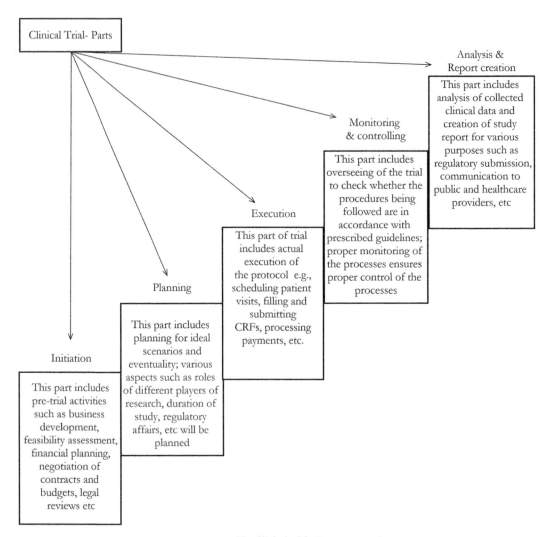

Fig: Clinical trial - Process overview

Some important aspects of trial process have been discussed in detail below:

5.11 Formulation of Research Question

An explicitly characterized and particular research question becomes a compelling component in decision making related to the different aspects of the study such as study design, population type, population size, type of data required to be collected and analysed.

The main challenges in developing an appropriate research question are:

(a)   to discover clinical uncertainties which could or should be examined and

(b)   to justify the need for that research

Researcher must understand what has been discovered and studied about the concerned topic till date. Before starting the trial, the researcher delves into all the available information which is related to the investigational product. This helps the researcher to develop a research question and the relevant objective.

It is a very important that the question and the objective of the trial are clearly specified before the trial starts. Thorough study of previously gathered information on the concerned topic spurs a number of questions which must be categorized as primary, secondary, etc at the beginning of the study. Primary question should always be given priority as it decides the basis of the hypothesis and study objectives.

Frameworks that helps in framing the research question are mentioned in the Fig – **Systems that aid in framing specifications of the research question**.

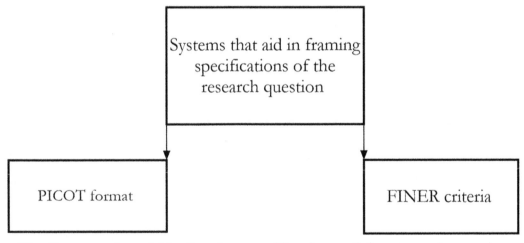

Fig: Systems that aid in framing specifications of the research question

5.12 PICOT and FINER frames

There are various approaches which can be used for the formulation of a research question. Out of these "the PICOT approach" is one of the most widely used approach (refer to the **Fig – PICOT**).

PICO(T)				
Patient/Population/ Problem	Intervention	Comparision	Outcome	Time(optional)
Which particular patient/ population/problem is the researcher interested in? Example: Women with normal pregnancy	What is investigational intervention (e.g. drug intervention, surgical, etc)? Example: Use of experimental drug X	What is the main alternative (reference/standard/ control) to compare with the investigational intervention? Example: Comparison with standard treatment drug Y	What is expected to accomplish through the study? Example: Increase in hemoglobin count	What will be the duration of data collection? Example: During Pregnancy

Fig: PICO(T)

Once the research question has been framed in accordance with the PICOT approach, the next step is to identify whether the research question meets the FINER criteria (refer to the **Fig – FINER criteria**).

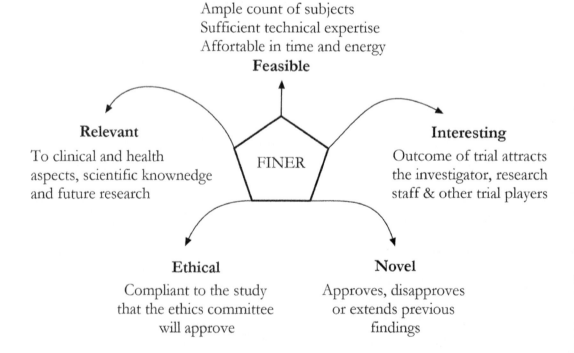

Fig: FINER Criteria

If the research question fulfils the needs of PICOT and FINER criteria, the researcher can finalize his/her research question.

5.13 Formulation of objectives and hypothesis

Post the selection of research question, the research objective and hypothesis need to be defined.

Research objective demonstrates what all the researcher expects to achieve through a proposed research. The research objectives can be considered as parts of an aim. The aims are statements which highlights what is needed to be achieved. It does not focus on how it has to be achieved. Thus, aim only concentrates on the outcomes which are desired from testing the hypotheses.

The objective of a research project should be "SMART" (refer to the **Fig – Characteristic of a research objective**).

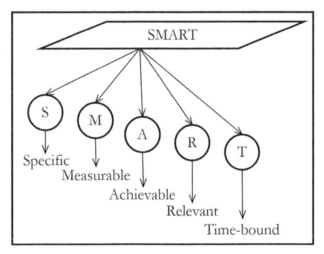

Fig: Characteristic of a research objective

A SMART objective helps in defining what exactly need to be done (specific) in a defined timeline (time bound) to achieve the aim of the research (relevant). It demonstrates that the target is achievable within the available research environment (achievable) and it also tracks/ measures the progress of the research (measurable).

The objective of a research must be very clear stated and it should be directly linked to the research question. Importance of research objective are listed in the **Fig – Importance of research objective.**

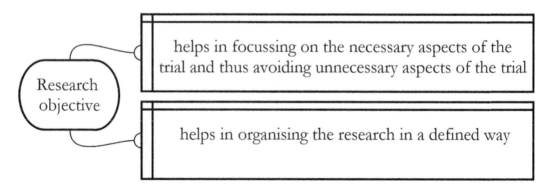

Fig: Importance of research objective

A study can have multiple objectives such as primary objective, secondary objective, etc. Research objective can be categorised into general and specific objectives (refer to the **Fig – Categories of research objective**).

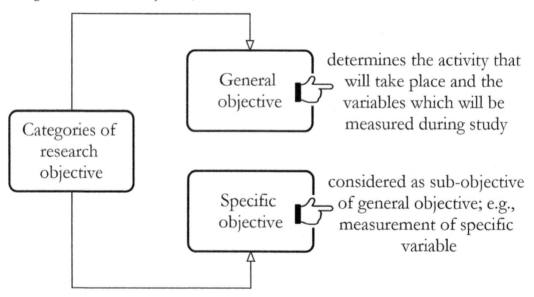

Fig: Categories of research objective

Research objectives can be defined through clear and precise statements which are called hypotheses. Hypotheses are possible answers to a research question. In other words, hypotheses are statements which a researcher makes about the potential outcome(s) of a study based on the research of literatures. It is a presumption on the basis of which a study has to be conducted. These hypotheses will be proved or disapproved on the basis of the outcomes of the proposed research.

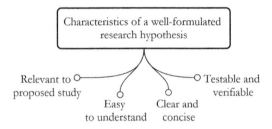

To develop research hypotheses, researcher need to identify a variable of a sample that causes or has an influence on another variable of the same/other sample.

5.14 Types of Variables

A variable is something that changes or we can say that a variable is an attribute or property of a person, event or object which is known to vary in a given study. It is a measurable characteristic of a person, an object or a phenomenon that can take on different values; e.g., individual's age. Different types of variables are depicted in the **Fig – Types of variables**.

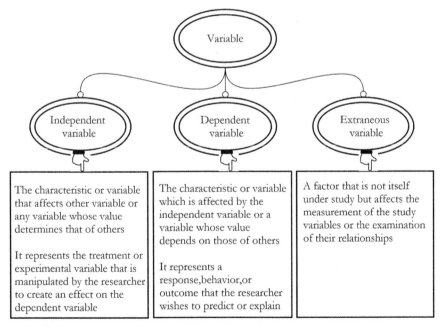

Fig: Types of variables

5.15 Ethics consideration

As it is obvious that the clinical trials involve human beings and it includes a direct intervention in human bodies, hence, it is paramount to take care of the ethical issues. The researcher may have collected some beneficial aspects from preclinical studies regarding the investigational product/treatment, but without a proper justification it is not possible to execute the clinical trials. Any medicinal product which has to be introduced amongst the general population, must be tested on the criteria of benefits and risks sufficiently and hence clinical trials are justified in this sense.

There are proper guidelines for conducting clinical trials or any research which involves human or any living body. The whole process of clinical trial takes place in accordance with the regulations. Every country has its own set of regulations for medical and clinical practices and the professionals who are working on an investigational product in humans in a country need to adhere to and follow the regulations of that particular country.

5.16 Target Population and sample population

Target population is the group of people within which the investigator identifies the result of his/her research, i.e. population in which findings of trial can be extrapolated. Once the target population is identified, the sample population need to be identified in which the experiment (intervention) can be done. Sample population should be representative of the target population (refer to the **Fig – Target population and Sample population**).

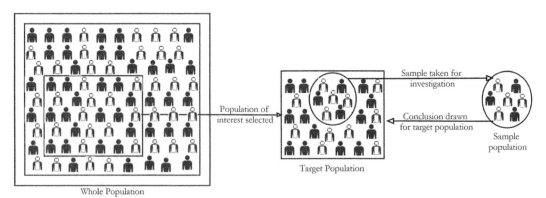

Fig: Target population and Sample population

5.17 Eligibility criteria

The sample population will pass through the eligibility (inclusion and exclusion) criteria (refer to the **Fig – Eligibility Criteria**) which may vary from trial to trial. Generally, the inclusion criteria include the patients who need investigative treatment and who will be benefitted from the investigation. Exclusion criteria, on the other hand excludes the individuals who can be put to a greater risk. Similarly, there are different factors (such as age, disease condition, duration of research, etc) which decide the inclusion and the exclusion of an interested participant in a particular trial.

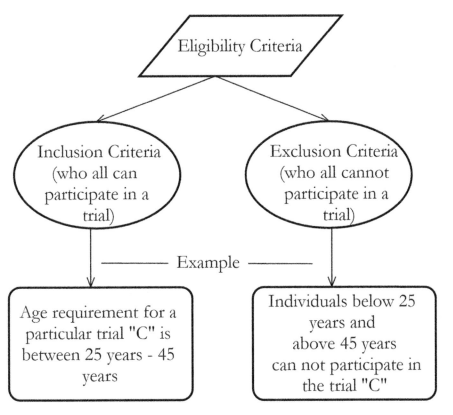

Fig: Eligibility Criteria

5.18 Informed Consent Process

The individuals eligible for trial are called for next step of the trial and this is the informed consent process, (refer to the **Fig – Informed Consent Process**).

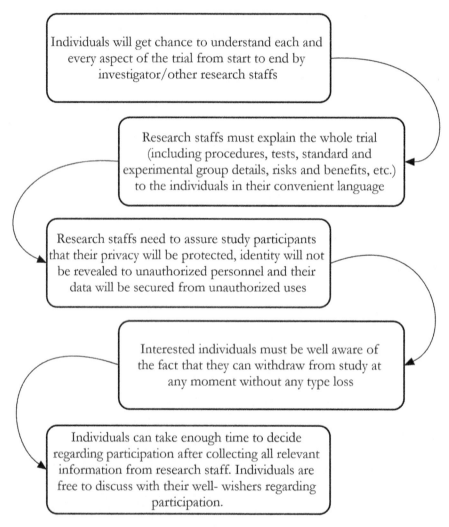

Fig: Informed Consent Process

Once the interested participants have completely understood and they are ready to participate voluntarily in the trial, they are required to sign the Informed Consent Form (ICF). Those participants who finally sign the ICF become a part of the study population (the population in which the trial will take place). Individuals who participate in a trial are called "Subjects".

5.19 Comparative studies Vs Non- comparative studies

In the event of non –comparative studies, it is hard to assess that till what extent the investigative medication has contributed to the patient's (who has been administered with investigative medication) improved condition, because there can be various factors (e.g. regular course of malady) which can compete for improvement of health.

Therefore, most of the clinical trials are comparative in nature. A comparative approach helps to study the effect of investigative intervention against the comparison group (refer to the **Fig – Typical comparative study design**). In a comparative study, the two groups (experimental group and placebo/control group) with subjects having similar characteristics are created so that the results at the end can provide a valid data i.e. any difference in the result would be due to the difference in intervention alone.

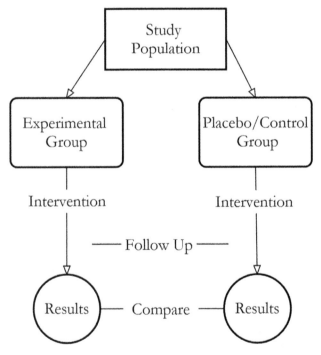

Fig: Typical comparative study design

The kind of treatment which is to be given to the control group (placebo or standard treatment), is a very important consideration. If an established treatment exists for the indication (which is being studied in the trial), then it will be unethical to use placebo. If standard treatment is used as a control, then it should be the best available option for the indication.

5.20 Placebo treatment

Placebo is a substance with no effects i.e. it does not contain active ingredients which are meant to affect health. Placebo looks like to be a "real" treatment but it is actually not a real treatment. Placebo could be a pill, distilled water, sugar or any other substance.

However, the use of Placebo can be rationalized in different medical conditions (refer to **Fig – Use of Placebo treatment**).

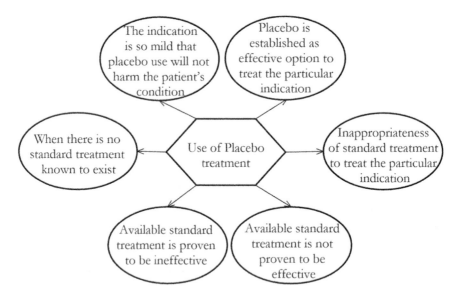

Fig: Use of Placebo treatment

Placebo is used during the studies to help the researcher to determine the effect of a new medicinal product for a particular indication. For instance, some of the participant may get the new drug for the target indication while some of the participants may get a placebo. At the end of the study, the researcher compares the effects of the drug and the placebo on the study participants. In this way, the researcher can establish the efficacy of the new drug.

Placebo effects, also known as Placebo response, can be due to direct or indirect causes (refer to **Fig – Causes of Placebo effects**).

5.21 Steps taken to avoid errors in clinical trial

There are numerous ways to create bias and variability in clinical trials which can impact the validity and integrity of the produced clinical data. Hence, it is important to take the steps in the trials which can minimize/eliminate these negative factors. Comparative study is one of the

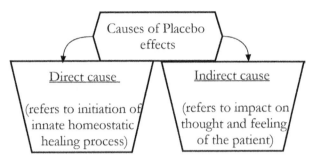

Fig: Causes of Placebo effects

step which is helpful to achieve valid results. Randomization and Blinding can also be helpful in minimizing/eliminating the errors in a trial.

5.22 Randomization

The investigator plays major role in a trial. All the decisions related to the trial pass through him/her. There are chances that the investigator becomes biased towards allocation of population into experimental or placebo/standard treatment. To avoid this probable malpractice, the random allocation of subjects can be done in the both groups (refer to the **Fig – Use of randomization in a clinical trial**). This method allows the allocation of study population on the basis of mere chance. Therefore, randomization helps to avoid the selection bias and it also helps to create the groups that are comparable in terms of distribution of known and unknown factors that may influence the outcome of the trial.

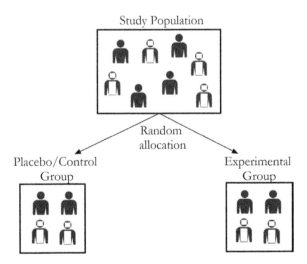

Fig: Use of randomization in a clinical trial

5.23 Blinding

It is possible that the response of the study population in a trial may get influenced if they become aware of the treatment they are getting. For instance, if the study subjects come to know that they are receiving placebo treatment, they will start feeling that there is no improvement.

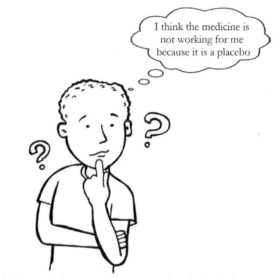

Study subject is aware of his treatment in a clinical trial
and he is thinking the medicine is not working because he
is getting placebo

Blinding (which is also known as masking) is done to avoid this kind of influencing effect where the patients are kept unaware of the treatment they would be receiving. This is called single blinding.

There are chances that the investigator may also end up in having an influenced response if he/she is aware of the treatments assignments in study subjects. In such cases, double blinding is required i.e. the investigator and patients, both are unaware of the treatment assignment.

In case of triple blinding the investigator, the patients and the data analyser, all are blinded with respect to the treatment assignment.

5.24 Monitoring compliance

The act of overseeing the progress of a clinical trial and ensuring that it is conducted, recorded, and reported in accordance with the protocol, standard operating procedures (SOPs), GCP, and the applicable regulatory requirement(s) is called "Monitoring".

Monitoring is a continuous quality control process during the entire clinical trial and it is generally performed by clinical research associate (CRA).

When a trial is conducted within the limits prescribed by the regulatory and legal authority, the trial is called compliant. The main objective of a controlled randomized trial is to elicit results from the intervention in ideal circumstances under a highly strict environment and regulations.

Monitoring compliance in a study is a very tough task for the research team. As there are many players involved in a trial, it is a big task to achieve and maintain perfect compliance in all aspect of the conduct of a trial. Trial without compliance will elicit imperfect and invalid results. Some examples of poor/noncompliance are mentioned in the **Fig – Examples of poor or noncompliance in a trial.**

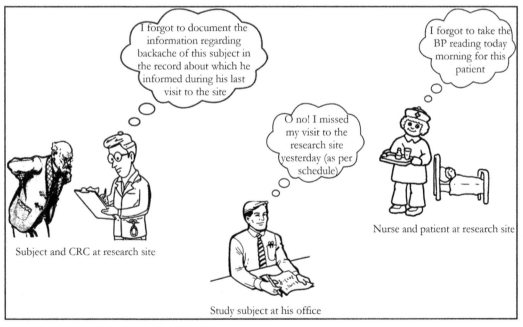

Fig: Examples of poor or noncompliance in a trial

Therefore, it is essential to keep a track of the level of compliance in the trial processes throughout the study. These tracking usually include maintaining self-report by subjects, proper follow up and accurate documentation by research personnel. There are many guidelines provided by the ethics committee and regulatory authority which are intended towards maintaining compliance in the trial.

5.25 Adverse events and safety monitoring

Subject safety is paramount in a trial. Hence, it is important that the protocol includes detailed instructions regarding collecting, assessing and reporting of the adverse events. Reporting on adverse events and the safety aspect during a trial is a very important job which needs to be performed by the investigator and CRC (Clinical Research Coordinator) very carefully and it should be done within the defined timelines. It must be done in a correct manner as it can impact many aspects including the results of a trial. It is mandatory for the investigator and the CRC to understand explicitly what to report, when to report, whom to report and how to report.

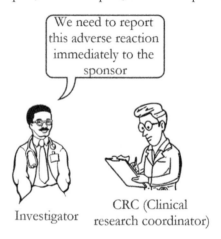

Fig: Investigator and CRC discussing about an
identified adverse reaction at the research site

There are a number of definitions related to the adverse event reporting and it is necessary to understand these definitions clearly and correctly. Example – it is important to understand the difference between the serious and the severe term in case of an event, because that will change the reporting criteria.

Most of the sponsors expect from the investigators that they report all serious adverse events that occur during a trial as soon as possible. This expectation is in order to ensure the safety of the subject and also to ease the regulatory requirements. In general, all non-serious adverse events will have to be recorded on a regular basis in CRF (Case Report Form) and the same will have to be reviewed and collected by CRA (Clinical Research Associate) during his/her visit to the site.

5.26 Clinical data management

Data management in a clinical trial is an integral part of the clinical studies (refer to the **Fig – Few processes of clinical data management**) as it ensures the validity, the quality and the integrity of data collected during trial from the subjects. A correctly handled clinical data management delivers a high-quality database for statistical analysis and which ultimately helps to draw conclusions regarding the safety and efficacy of the investigational product.

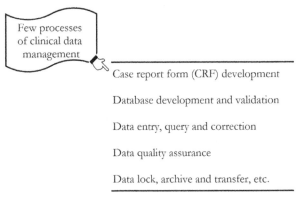

Case report form (CRF) development

Database development and validation

Data entry, query and correction

Data quality assurance

Data lock, archive and transfer, etc.

Fig: Few processes of clinical data management

5.27 Analysis of clinical data

Biostatistics is a branch of statistics which deals with the study of biological sciences. Biostatistics basically deals with variations arising out of the biological phenomena (refer to the **Fig – Uses of biostatistics in biological science field**). Example – Blood pressure varies within the normal range in a person and these slight changes in a single person at different point of time

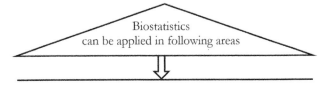

To decide endpoint(s) for a clinical trial

To estimate appropriate sample size for a trial

To analyse the clinical data produced during a clinical trial

To study the connection between two (or more) variables

To explain a given set of data (Descriptive biostatistics), etc

Fig: Uses of biostatistics in biological science field

can be considered normal (up to certain limit and within a certain range). In the similar way, there are other biological variations such as weight which can be looked in combination with the height, serum creatinine level, sugar level etc. among individuals which may occur due to different reasons and these are required to be studied for research and healthcare purpose.

In case, in a trial, all the subjects complete the full-length participation in accordance with compliance, and all other players also play their respective roles by being compliant, it will be easy to calculate the result of a trial. But generally, it does not happen in such an ideal manner as some incomplete cases exist in trial due to which it provides incomplete data. There are guidelines to handle such scenarios in the trial analysis. The two main approaches for analysis of clinical data are mentioned in the **Fig – Approaches to analyze clinical data**.

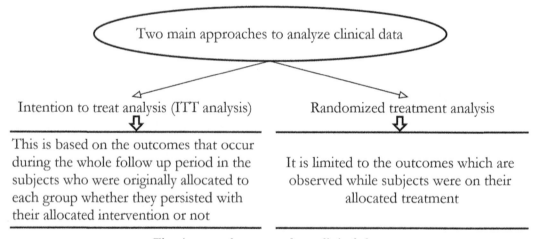

Fig: Approaches to analyze clinical data

However, ITT analysis is the correct way of analysing data.

5.28 ITT Analysis

Intention-to-treat (ITT) includes all randomized patients in the groups to which they were randomly assigned, regardless of their adherence with the entry criteria, regardless of the treatment they actually received, and regardless of subsequent withdrawal from treatment or deviation from the protocol [(Fisher *et al.* (1990)].

Although, RCT is considered the best method for the investigation, it also encounters different kinds of problem. Two main problems concerning RCT are mentioned in the **Fig – Problems encountered in RCT**.

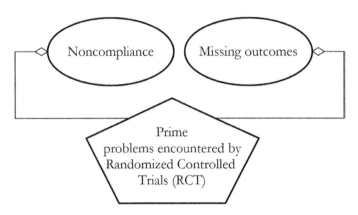

Fig: Problems encountered in RCT

ITT analysis provides a solution for the problems faced in RCT. ITT analysis considers that noncompliance and protocol deviations are likely to happen even in actual clinical practices. Hence, it includes all the study subjects (by ignoring noncompliance, protocol deviations, withdrawal, and anything that happens after randomization) during analysis to maintain the prognostic balance generated from the original random treatment allocation (refer to **Fig – Key feature of ITT analysis**). Therefore, it gives a fair estimate of treatment effect and it also represents the practical clinical scenario.

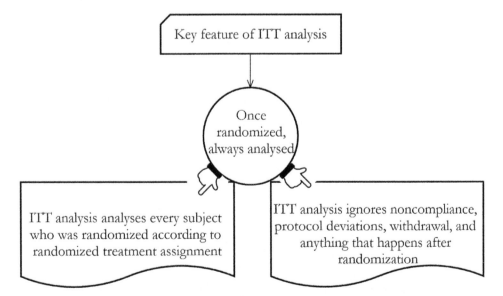

Fig: Key feature of ITT analysis

It is always better to analyze the data on a regular basis on its accumulation. It will give an idea about the progress or the gaps (if any) in the trial and will also save time at the end of the trial. An independent department is supposed to take care of the analysis part of the trial. These departments can suggest stopping or can even recommend changes in the trial if they find that there are any safety concerns for the subjects.

The analysis of data inspects if the randomization process has created balance of the baseline characteristics between/among the groups and that the two groups are comparable for final results. If all the subjects are recruited and followed up in the same period, the analysis can be done to compare the effects in the different groups. However, in many trials, the recruitment goes on for several years and thus the details related to follow up and intervention duration for subjects vary.

5.29 RCT (Randomized Controlled Trial) – Introduction

RCT is type of clinical trial/study where the participants are randomly (by chance) assigned to one of two (or more) treatment group. The treatment groups are similar in all respects except in their interventions which are decided by randomization. (refer to the **Fig – RCT stands for Randomized Controlled Trial**).

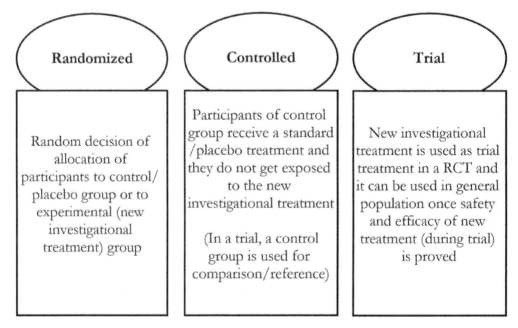

Fig: RCT stands for Randomized Controlled Trial

5.30 Features of RCT

RCT is considered a "Gold standard" for evaluating the effectiveness of new medical interventions. Important features of RCT are listed in the **Fig – Features of RCT**.

RCT is the most rigorous way of determining if a cause-effect relation exists between the treatment and the outcome i.e. it determines if the intervention itself, as opposed to other factors, causes the observed outcome

The main aim of randomization is to ensure that any observed differences between the treatment groups exist only due to the differences in the treatment alone and not due to the effects of confounding (known or unknown) factors or bias.

RCT is a very helpful method in assessing the cost effectiveness of a treatment

---

Fig: Features of RCT

For fair results in the trial, the factors (e.g., age, sex, weight, ethnicity, etc.) within the participants of the control group should be in matching with the factors within the participants of the experimental group. Control group may receive placebos (dummy treatments). Ethical or practical perspectives need to be considered while using a placebo (such as declining treatment to people who have a life-threatening or serious illness).

5.31 Basic structure of RCT

In a RCT design, two groups are formed i.e.:

(a)   the experimental group (which receives investigational treatment) and

(b)   the control group (which receives standard/placebo treatment)

A sample (out of population of interest) is taken and divided randomly into experimental group and control group. Both the groups (which are supposed to have received different interventions) are treated and observed in an identical manner and they are followed up for a specified period of time (refer to the **Fig – Basic structure of RCT**).

At the end of the study, all the data collected during the study from control group and experimental group are analysed and compared. The difference in the outcomes can be attributed to the new intervention because both the groups were treated identically except that there are different interventions.

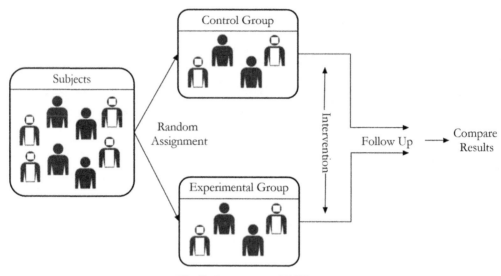

Fig: Basic structure of RCT

5.32 Importance of RCT

Randomized Controlled Trial (RCT) has been established as the most reliable and unbiased tool for hypothesis testing as it provides a powerful form of evidence for medical practices (refer to the **Fig – Importance of RCT**).

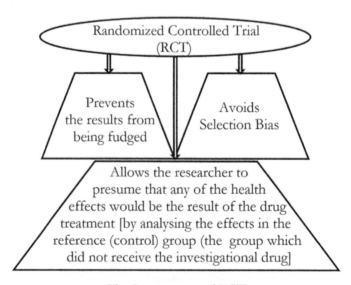

Fig: Importance of RCT

Selection bias is the selection of individuals, groups or data for analysis in such a way that it does not lead to achieving of proper randomization, thereby ensuring that the sample obtained is not representative of the population intended to be analysed. It is sometimes referred to as the selection effect.

Example – In a non-randomized trial, suppose that a researcher is trying to show that the investigational product is more effective, he/she may not expose certain patients to the experimental product by estimating that investigational product may produce bad effects, thus establishing an experimental product look more beneficial overall than it may be in reality. Similarly, if researcher is trying to establish that an investigational product is not effective, they may expose patients with a higher risk of complications to the investigational product.

5.33 Commonly used designs in RCT

Randomized controlled trial (RCT) can be done with various designs depending upon (a) the availability of the study subjects, (b) the type of indication being studied, (c) the duration of study, (d) the phase of trial, etc. Some common designs used in RCT are listed in the **Fig – Types of designs used in RCT**.

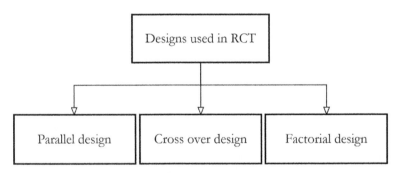

Fig: Types of designs used in RCT

5.34 Parallel design

- A parallel designed clinical trial compares the results of treatments in two separate groups of patients. Usually an investigational treatment is compared with a standard treatment.

- The subjects are randomized to two (or more) treatment groups called the experimental group and the control group and both the groups receive the respective treatment till the end of the trial (refer to the **Fig – Parallel Design**)

- Important features of Parallel design are described in the **Fig – Features of Parallel design**.

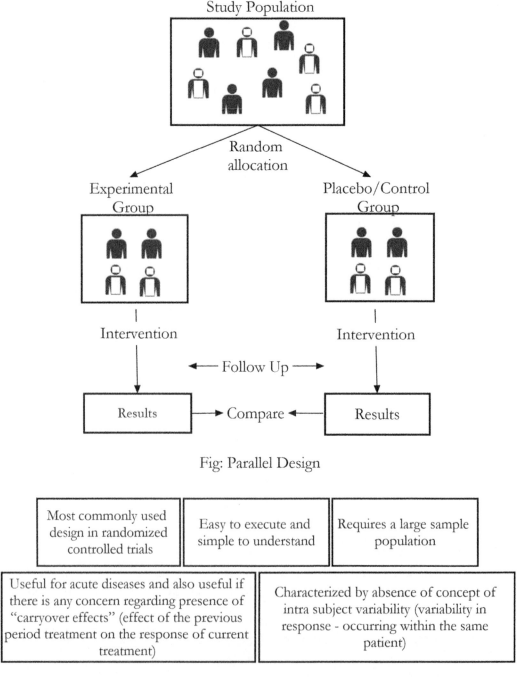

Fig: Parallel Design

Most commonly used design in randomized controlled trials	Easy to execute and simple to understand	Requires a large sample population

Useful for acute diseases and also useful if there is any concern regarding presence of "carryover effects" (effect of the previous period treatment on the response of current treatment)	Characterized by absence of concept of intra subject variability (variability in response - occurring within the same patient)

Fig: Features of Parallel design

5.35 Cross over design

- Cross over design is a trial in which both the groups receive both treatments (standard/ placebo and experimental) but at different time. At a predefined time in the trial, one group switches from control treatment to experimental treatment and the other group switches from experimental treatment to control treatment

- Some terms which are used in cross over design are mentioned below:

- Sequence - Order of treatment administration in a crossover experiment

- Period - Time of a treatment administration

- Capital letters are used to denote treatments such as A, B, etc.

- Wash out period – time between treatment periods

- The most popular crossover design 2 × 2 crossover design: 2-sequences (AB and BA), 2-periods, 2-treatments

- In this particular design, subjects are randomized to sequence AB and sequence BA (refer to the **Fig – Cross over design**).

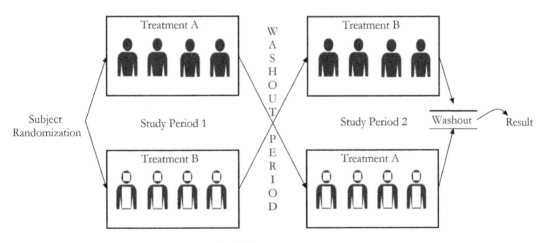

Fig: Cross-over design

- The subjects in sequence AB receive treatment A in the first period and treatment B in the second period, whereas subjects in sequence BA receive treatment B in the first period and treatment A in the second period. It can be represented as follows:

	Period 1	Period 2
Sequence AB	A	B
Sequence BA	B	A

- Important features of Cross over design are mentioned in the **Fig – Features of Cross over design.**

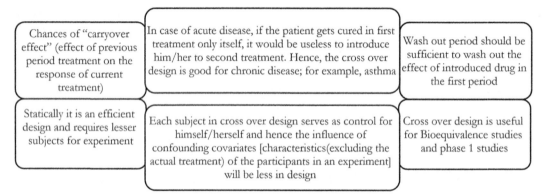

Fig: Features of Cross over design

5.36 Comparative study of Parallel and Cross-over design

Features	Parallel Design	Cross-over Design
Treatment assignment	Group of subjects are assigned different (standard or experimental) treatments	Each of the subject is assigned to both (standard and experimental) treatment
Sample size	Large	Small
Duration	Shorter	Longer
Carryover effects	No	Yes
Used for	Acute diseases	Chronic diseases

5.37 Factorial Design

- Factorial design helps to evaluate two or more questions simultaneously in one trial

- It saves time and needs fewer subjects to study two or more factors

- 2^*2 is the most common design but it is seldom used

- In 2*2 design - the participants are randomized to treatment A and the corresponding placebo to test one hypothesis and then they are randomized again to treatment B and the corresponding placebo to study the second hypothesis. This enables the study of two different hypotheses simultaneously. This design can be depicted as follows:

Treatment B & Corresponding Placebo	Treatment A & Corresponding Placebo		
		Placebo	Treatment A
	Placebo	Neither A or B	A only
	Treatment B	B only	Both A and B

- It is important to avoid interaction between the two treatments i.e. treatment A and treatment B because the interaction between two treatments can complicate the interpretation of effects of treatment however, the study of interaction would be important if the treatments are meant to be used together

Other designs include Adaptive trial design, Randomized withdrawal approach, Superiority, Non- inferiority, etc.

Chapter 6

CLINICAL TRIAL – OPERATIONAL ASPECTS

6.1 Learnings from the chapter

- *Various aspects of clinical trial such as investigator identification, site identification, basic infrastructure, approvals, funds for research, meetings, etc.*

- *Ethics committee and their contribution in a trial*

- *Types of agreements and types of files used in a trial*

- *Trial close out and record retention details*

- *SOP details*

6.2 Introduction

All research involving human participants require approval from a Research Ethics Committee prior to starting of any study procedures. Once the required approval is obtained from the authorities, the trial/study steps can be initiated. Operational aspects of a clinical trial start with investigator identification.

6.3 Investigator identification

Sponsors identify an investigator suitable for their study mainly with three traits (refer to the **Fig – Traits of Investigator**).

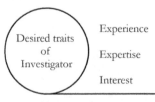

Fig: Traits of Investigator

Investigator selection is mainly dependent on the requirements of the study protocol. Investigators need to submit their Curriculum Vitae (CV) to the sponsor so that the sponsor can get an idea about investigator's qualification, research activities and other important aspects which is mandatory to run a successful trial. Conversing with the investigator is also very helpful in exploring the investigator's interest in the respective trial. Most often, the Clinical Research Associate (CRA) plays representative role of sponsor at research site.

FDA maintains a list of debarred Investigators and displays the list on its website. Sponsor must go through it before finalizing any investigator. Other sources such as colleagues in medical field, who may be knowing the investigator, can be referred to regarding selection of investigator.

6.4 Site identification

Site selection is another important criterion for successful completion of a trial. Clinical research associate (CRA) visits the site to ensure that all required elements (Refer to **Fig – Aspects checked during site identification**) for a trial are present at the prospective site. Prior to CRA visit, investigator and other research staff should read the protocol thoroughly so that they can make a clear conversation with CRA about the upcoming trial to the site.

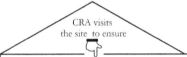

CRA visits
the site to ensure

Site facilities - adequate for trial purpose

Site staff - well qualified and trained and sufficient in number to run the trial

Stability of site staff in their jobs - important fot smooth operation of trial (long tenure of staff creates good relationship with subjects which results in comfortable environment for subjects and their retention till the end of trial)

Availability of storage solutions - to store trial related supplied materials

Availability of equipment -enough to perform the trial

Feasibility of site - for potential enrollment

Ongoing and competitive studies details (if any)

Timing of trial - suitable for site staff (site staff should be able to concentrate on the trial with other site activities)

Laboratory and Pharmacy facilities - important to ensure production of valid data during trial

Location of site - convenient for CRA and the participants for regular visits

Vendor management - adequately planned

Availability of site management organization(SMO) - if required to manage compliance, relevant data capture and transcription in defined timeline

Fig: Aspects checked during site identification

6.5 Basic Infrastructure

CRA visits the site to estimate the suitability of the site for the trial. He or she evaluates the space available for the study and to ascertain on how these will be used for the trial. There are different aspects of trial which may demand individual space. Some of the important spaces are described in **Fig – Basic Infrastructure**.

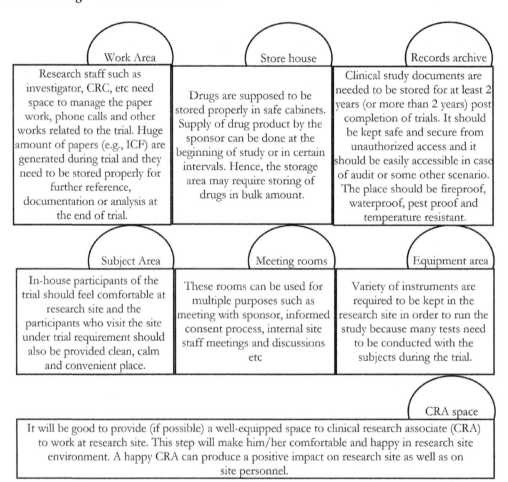

Fig: Basic Infrastructure

6.6 Source documents

A source document refers to the original documents, data and records where information is first captured. Some examples of source documents are hospital records, clinical and office charts, laboratory notes, etc. Information from these data are usually captured and transcribed onto the Case Report Form (CRF). Sometimes, the original data is collected directly in the patient diary or CRF; in such cases, these documents become the source document.

It is important to review source document throughout the study. This process examines many important aspects of the trial (refer to the **Fig – Importance of source document verification**). This process of review is known as "source document verification or source document review". Clinical research associate (CRA) takes the responsibility of the source document verification.

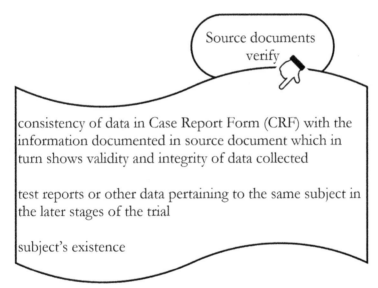

Fig: Importance of source document verification

It is important to keep the source document available during the CRA visit whenever the visit happens for source document verification and also for verifying compliance with respect to the other study requirements.

6.7 Ethics committee – IRBs/IECs

The International Council on Harmonisation (ICH) defines an institutional review board (IRB) as a group, formally designated to protect the rights, safety and well-being of humans involved in a clinical trial by reviewing all the aspects of the trial and by approving its start up. IRBs can also be called independent ethics committees (IECs). Ethics Committee is an independent body constituted of people from medical/science background and non-medical/non-scientific background.

6.8 Types of IRBs/IECs

IRBs/IECs can be local or central (refer to the **Fig – Types of IRBs/IECs**) depending upon their association and functions.

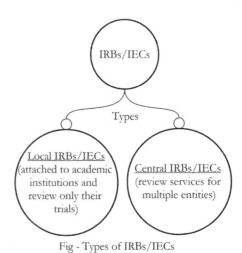

Fig - Types of IRBs/IECs

6.9 Need for Ethics Committee

Prior to enrollment of volunteers in a trial, IEC/IRB must review all study related materials. IRB/IEC also does periodic reviews called "continuing reviews" throughout the trial. (Continuing reviews may take place at least once a year and include the entire trial along with the changes made.).

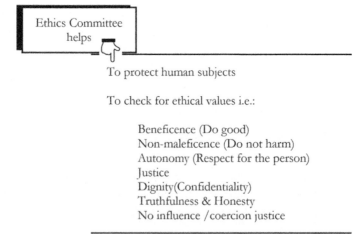

To protect human subjects

To check for ethical values i.e.:

Beneficence (Do good)
Non-maleficence (Do not harm)
Autonomy (Respect for the person)
Justice
Dignity(Confidentiality)
Truthfulness & Honesty
No influence /coercion justice

6.10 Responsibilities of IRB/IEC

The IRB/IEC review ensures that all the ethical aspects in the proposed research are maintained properly and it also ensures that the proposed research is scientifically sound. Some of the important roles of IEC/IRB are listed in **Fig – Roles of IRB/IEC**.

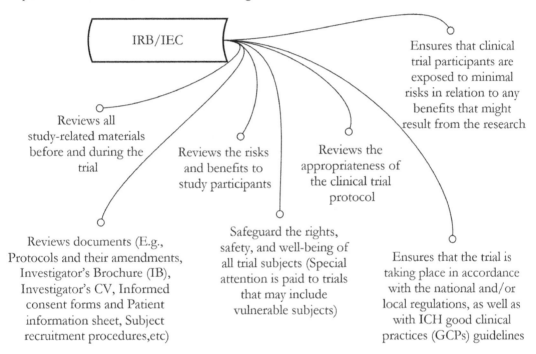

IRB/IEC

Ensures that clinical trial participants are exposed to minimal risks in relation to any benefits that might result from the research

Reviews all study-related materials before and during the trial

Reviews the risks and benefits to study participants

Reviews the appropriateness of the clinical trial protocol

Reviews documents (E.g., Protocols and their amendments, Investigator's Brochure (IB), Investigator's CV, Informed consent forms and Patient information sheet, Subject recruitment procedures,etc)

Safeguard the rights, safety, and well-being of all trial subjects (Special attention is paid to trials that may include vulnerable subjects)

Ensures that the trial is taking place in accordance with the national and/or local regulations, as well as with ICH good clinical practices (GCPs) guidelines

Fig - Roles of IRB/IEC

It is good to be aware of the ethics committee and their various activity timelines such as their meeting frequency, the time taken for approval process, etc. All this information will be helpful for the researchers to estimate the time consumption in the regulation processes.

It is the responsibility of the principal investigator (PI) to ensure that conduct of the trial is compliant with IRB/IEC requirements. PI may deviate from the study protocol without prior IRB/IEC approval only to eliminate immediate safety hazard to a study participant. But, PI must notify the IRB/IEC of any deviations which may arise from the protocol as soon as possible.

6.11 Ongoing studies and Competitive studies

CRA must make a note of all the ongoing studies including competitive studies (if any) and the usual clinical practices going on at the site, as these can decide the availability of investigator and other research staffs for an upcoming project. It is good to check the details of competitive studies that can compete for same subject pool requirement because that can impact the subject recruitment rate for upcoming trial.

6.12 Agreements

If any third party (including commercial, facilities or services provider) is involved in the trial, then the contracts and agreements need to be executed in the beginning or prior to start of the trial. Examples of service providers may include supplier of the medical products (such as device), funders, laboratory and pharmacy services providers and others.

An agreement is a concord of understanding and intention between two or more parties, with respect to the effect upon their relative rights and duties of certain past or future facts or performances.

There are number of agreements used in a clinical trial. Some of those are explained in the **Fig – Types of Agreements**.

Confidentiality Disclosure Agreement (CDA)	
an agreement type which is usually the first agreement between the sponsor and the investigator or vendor/service providers before sharing of protocol/ IB or other confidential documents. It is also known as non- disclosure/confidentiality agreement.	
Registry Agreement (RA) an agreement that governs situations in which patients are required to provide informed consent to have their health information recorded in a registry database	**Clinical Trial Agreement (CTA)** an agreement governing the terms and obligations of all parties during the conduct of a clinical trial. This agreement must be fully executed prior to study activation.
Protocol Agreement an agreement which indicates the investigator's consent to conduct the trial as per the protocol.	**FDA Form 1572** an agreement signed by the investigator to ensure that he/she will comply with FDA regulations related to the conduct of trial for an investigational product
Data Use Agreement (DUA) an agreement that governs the transfer of data outside the context of a CTA or Sponsored Research Agreement (SRA).	**Financial Agreement** an agreement which details about the payments to the investigator and /or institute per subject in the study.

Fig: Types of Agreements

Other agreements include vendor agreements such as agreement for Site Management Organization, Investigational product management, Contract research organization (CRO), etc.

6.13 Financial Disclosures

According to Code of Federal Regulations (CFR), Title 21, Part 54, financial disclosure is a required item in the conduct of a trial. FDA demands from the applicant the submission of a list of all clinical investigators who conducted clinical studies and to identify those who are full-time or part-time employees of the sponsor for each of the study. For each clinical investigator who was not a full-time or part-time employee of a sponsor of the clinical study, the applicant has to provide a certification (either using form FDA 3454 or using form FDA 3455).

Thus, according to Federal Regulations, clinical Investigators are required to disclose to the sponsor their financial interests for the period of time he/she participated in the study and for one year following the end of his/her participation in the study (refer to the **Fig – Financial interest and disclosure**).

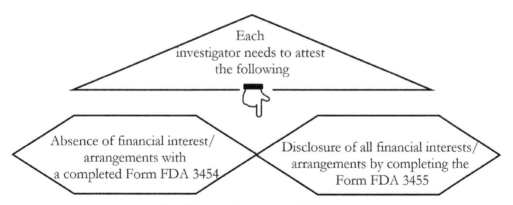

Fig: Financial interest and disclosure

Financial disclosures must be collected at the start of the trial. Financial disclosures ensure that financial interests and arrangements of clinical investigators that could affect the reliability of data submitted to FDA are identified and disclosed by the applicant. FDA may consider (a) size and nature of disclosed financial interest (b) the potential increase in the value of interest, in case the investigational product gets approval and (c) the steps that have been taken to minimize the potential for bias.

In case of any changes to these financial disclosures, the investigator must update the status of the financial disclosure during the study period and it should continue till one-year post study completion.

Having a financial interest in a company or a product cannot be the reason for not taking that investigator for the trial. Financial disclosures just make the information available to all the parties about the potential for conflict of interest.

6.14 Approvals

To conduct a clinical trial, it is imperative to get the required approvals from the regulatory authorities. In the process of getting approval for a particular trial, a Clinical Trial Application will be required to be submitted to the regulatory body. Research Ethics Committee (REC) will also participate in the review process of the same trial and provides its opinion on the proposed research.

These reviews are done to ensure that the dignity, rights, safety and well-being of the study subjects are respected and protected in the trial. Clinical trials are typically conducted at universities, hospitals, or clinics. Post the required approval, the trial is closely monitored by the ethics committee.

Although, national legislation decides the duties of ethics committee, certain internationally recognized common features are set for every ethics committees (example -assessment and review of all types of human research is one of the responsibilities of ethics committee).

Clinical trials must be conducted in compliance with regulations, ethical principles and prescribed guidelines. Standards of ICH-GCP must be applied and maintained in the trial.

6.15 Funds for research

There can be many sources from where the researchers can get funds for their research. A research can be funded by multiple funders and/or multiple sponsors. An independent organisation (a sponsor) can also fund a research. Funders should be contacted at the earliest in the planning stage of the clinical trial.

The funding application should be appropriately priced, and then the costs and payments involved in the trial process should be identified. Few examples of costs related to a trial are mentioned in the **Fig – Examples of costs.**

6.16 Investigator meetings

These meetings are organized by the sponsor for multicentre trial (a trial which involve several sites but same protocol) however, these meetings are not required by the regulations. The purpose of these meetings is to ensure safe and effective execution of the study protocol.

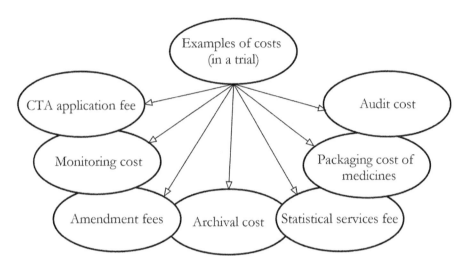

Fig: Examples of costs (in a trial)

Timing and venue of these meetings should be such that it ensures maximum attendance because these meetings can help in enhancing the performance of the research staff and in producing quality data. Important features related to Investigator meetings are mentioned in the **Fig – Features of Investigator meetings**.

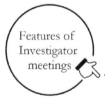

These meetings include all investigators, coordinators and appropriate sponsor representative(s)

These meetings create opportunities for all the parties and staff to know each other in advance, which in turn helps in smooth communication throughout the study

These meetings are one of the important activities pertaining to conduct of a good trial because these meetings train investigator and other research staff on trial related activities and applicable regulations

Most favourable time for conducting these meetings is just before the trial initiation as every staff would be fresh with respect to the information discussed in meeting

Fig: Features of Investigator meetings

These meetings provide information related to the different aspects of the trial (refer to the **Fig – Topics included in Investigator meetings**). Hence, proper preparation for the meeting can be helpful for the investigator and clinical research coordinator (CRC) as they can clarify their doubts (if any) in the meeting.

Investigator meetings include the following topics

Discussion of study protocol which includes investigator responsibilities, trial processes, outcomes, etc

Regulatory and IEC/IRB requirements

CRF related guidelines (in detail) and safety reporting

CRA visits details, SOPs, Source documentation, etc.

Fig: Topics included in Investigator meetings

6.17 Initiation Meetings

Initiation meetings, also known as "start-up visit" occur at the research site post obtaining all the required regulatory approvals. All study related materials are supplied to the site and the recruitment process is then expected to start. Important features related to Initiation meetings are mentioned in **Fig – Features of Initiation meetings**.

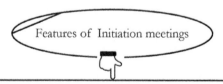

Features of Initiation meetings

These meetings create opportunities to train all the research staff on the procedures and on the other aspects related to the study

Agenda of these meetings are similar to the investigator meeting but initiation meetings can have a detailed review of safety reporting guidelines, GCP compliance, CRF completion guidelines, etc.

Most often, the CRA is responsible for initiation meetings and it is important for all the staffs to attend these meetings as the attendance and documentation of training is essential to fulfil the regulatory requirement of training research staffs

Fig: Features of Initiation meetings

The purpose of an initiation meeting is to ensure that the investigators and other research staff understand the study protocol properly. It also ensures that everyone is clear and well trained in their specific roles and responsibilities. Sponsors do not allow to start trial before occurrence of these meetings. Post initiation meeting, site can start enrolment of subjects.

6.18 Comparative study of Investigator meetings and Initiation meetings

Features	Investigator meetings	Initiation meetings
Purpose	To train the members of all study sites (in case of multicenter study) regarding the different aspects of the particular trial and regulatory requirements	To train the members of the individual study site regarding the different aspects of the particular trial and regulatory requirements
Place of meetings	In desired location such as a hotel or hall	At the research site
Discussion topics	Different aspects of the study protocol, CRFs, safety reporting, SOPs, regulatory requirements, etc.	Different aspects of the study protocol, CRFs, safety reporting, SOPs, regulatory requirements, etc.
Who all participate?	All principal investigators, CRCs and representatives of the Sponsor/CRO of all sites of a study	Principal investigator, CRC, other site staff and representatives of the Sponsor/CRO of an individual site of a study
When to take place?	Close to the start of the enrolment process	Immediately before patient recruitment is expected to start

{Recruitment and retention of the volunteers - Refer to chapter 9 – Human participation in a Clinical trial (research)

Adverse event reporting - Refer to chapter 11 – Safety monitoring of a therapeutic product}

6.19 Trial/study files

Proper filing of study documents at the research site is required to run the trial in a hassle-free manner. A trial contains variety of documents which can be categorized as clinical files, administrative files and regulatory files (refer to the **Fig – Categories of trial/study files**).

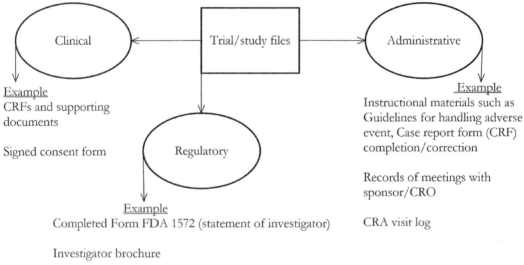

Example
CRFs and supporting
documents

Signed consent form

Example
Instructional materials such as
Guidelines for handling adverse
event, Case report form (CRF)
completion/correction

Records of meetings with
sponsor/CRO

Example
Completed Form FDA 1572 (statement of investigator)   CRA visit log

Investigator brochure

Original written IRB approvals of the study protocol and
consent form

Signed original copy of protocol and amendments

Copies of the laboratory certification and normal ranges

Investigational New Drug (IND) application

Fig: Categories of trial/study files

There can be many reasons (e.g., audit, emergency, avoiding loss of information) behind the requirement to maintain study files at the site. Hence, it is important for the research staff to understand how to maintain the trial related documents in an appropriate manner. The research staff can ask for help from CRA in understanding the methods of maintaining the trial related documents at the site.

Ideally, the study files should be set up at the site before starting the trial. CRA needs to review the document maintenance processes periodically throughout the trial period. Files should be easily accessible whenever required (for example – at the time of visit of CRA). But, it is also imperative to keep the files secured from unauthorized persons. For example, if a site is conducting more than one trial for different sponsors, then it is mandatory for investigators to ensure that CRA of one of the sponsor does not get access to the documents of another sponsor's trial.

Once the trial is over, all the documents related to the trial should be kept in proper way so that the documents are easily accessible as the documents have to be made available for further review, reference, audit, etc. Some methods like coloured stickers, stamp, etc can be used to mark the charts and materials of study subject for easy access and identification. Several companies are using electronic trial master file which can save time, space and environment as well.

6.20 Storage and Dispensing of Investigational product

According to ICH-GCP, all involved parties (e.g., site monitor, investigator, pharmacist) in a trial must be well informed about the handling of investigational product [e.g., storage condition, route of administration, procedures and devices for product infusion (if any)]. Sponsor plays an important role in handling of the investigational product (refer to the **Fig – Sponsor's responsibilities towards investigational product**).

Sponsor needs to

To communicate properly to research staff regarding handling of investigational product

To control the distribution of investigational product and to ensure that investigational product is shipped only to the trial investigator

To maintain proper documentation of receipt, shipment or other disposition of investigational product

To check the return of all unused materials from the research site

Fig: Sponsor's responsibilities towards investigational product

Care should be taken in the administration of investigational product as the trial product should be administered only to the trial subjects. This drug administration should be done under supervision of investigator or sub-investigator. Access to the product must be limited to authorized persons only. There can be many issues regarding the handling of the investigational product. Some of the problems are mentioned in **Fig – Problems identified with investigational product**.

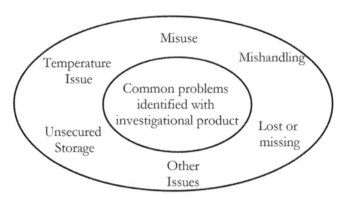

Fig: Problems identified with the investigational product

Records related to handling of investigational product must be updated on time otherwise it can lead to mismanagement of investigational product.

6.21 Trial close out

When a study is completed at an investigative site, the site should be closed officially. Study close out procedure starts with database locking. The close out process includes closing out of different sites of a trial (in case of multicentre trial), collection of all trial files, reconciliation and destruction of investigational product and notification to ethics committees and regulatory agencies. Once the data is analysed, interpreted and clinical study report is prepared, the prepared report can be distributed to different sites, ethics committees and regulatory authorities.

Closure procedure

Investigator makes everything ready with the help of clinical research coordinator (CRC) before CRA visits the research site for the closure procedure of the trial. To ensure the proper completion of closeout procedure, CRA examines the different aspects of the trial thoroughly (refer to the **Fig – Closure procedure**).

CRA ensures that completion of final report is done in an appropriate manner. This final report includes enrolment summary, dropout details, detail of adverse events and trial relevant other details. Copies of this report will be submitted to IRB and sponsor.

6.22 Record retention

Record retention must happen according to the regulations. Regulations require each investigator to retain research data not only while the research is being conducted but also after the research is completed. There should be documented procedures in place which define (a) the processes for archiving the trial records and materials, (b) the checks for completeness, (c) timeframes for

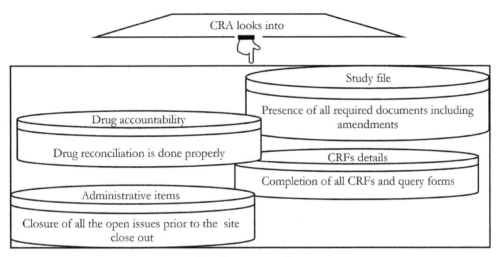

Fig: Closure procedure

submission to archive, (d) delegation of responsibility for submission of record and material to the archive, etc. There are several different regulations each of which has different requirements (refer to the **Fig – Regulations for record retention**).

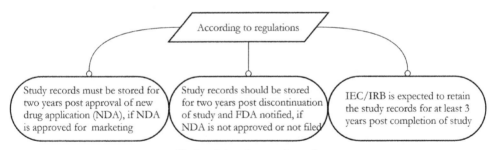

Fig: Regulations for record retention

The archival location of the records must be clearly mentioned and should be easily accessible for audit or inspection purpose. Sponsor suggests investigator to store the study records in good condition so that if sponsor wishes to file a new application based on an old study, the old study records would be helpful for FDA review. In most of the cases, sponsor provides place to store study records safely till the time all processes are completed.

6.23 Reasons for study closure

On the completion of study, the study closure is normal but sometimes, the study can be closed early (before set duration). The various favourable or unfavourable reasons for study closure are mentioned in the **Fig – Reasons for study closure**.

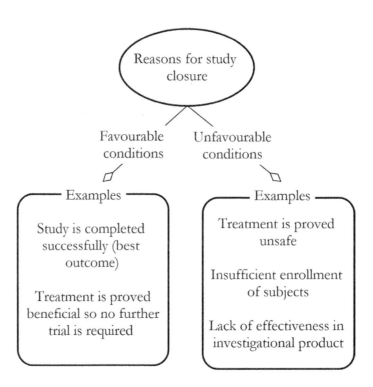

Fig: Reasons for study closure

In case of termination of study before set time, the sponsor has to make sure that all investigators and research staffs are well informed about the steps that need to be taken for study subjects. Research staffs need to assure the subjects about their treatment and follow-up processes post trial termination.

6.24 Standard Operating Procedures (SOPs)

SOPs are important to standardize the processes and procedures involved in a trial. SOPs ensure that all the research staffs are well aware of the correct way to perform their assigned tasks. SOPs also ensure that all the regulations and good clinical practices are followed during the trial.

SOPs are written procedures prescribed for repetitive use as practice in accordance with agreed upon specifications aimed at obtaining a desired outcome. SOPs explain how to perform a particular task.

SOPs are required to be followed by all the players such as investigative sites, ethics committee, sponsor for a successful completion of trial (refer to the **Fig – Benefits of SOPs**).

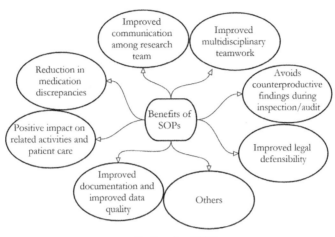

Fig: Benefits of SOPs

Once the SOPs and guidelines are ready for a particular trial, it is very important to train all involved personnel in trial about SOPs and guidelines, otherwise the SOPs will be of no use if they are not implemented properly in the trial system. SOPs and guidelines are supposed to be reviewed at least annually to ensure that it continues to be relevant and workable. If it is not so, then the changes must be updated in all the documents where all staffs can access them. All changes must be well documented for audit purpose.

In a clinical trial, different types of SOPs are prepared (refer to the **Fig – Different types of SOPs prepared in clinical trials**).

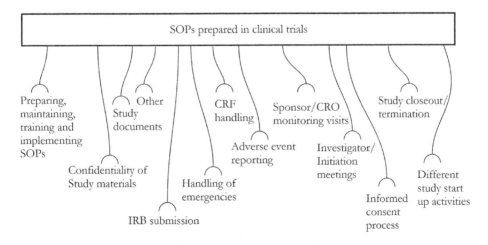

Fig: Different types of SOPs prepared in clinical trials

Chapter 7

RESEARCH PROTOCOL

7.1 Learnings from the chapter

- *Protocol definition and its approval*

- *Key elements of protocol and protocol preparation*

- *Need and importance of research protocol and its different users*

- *Types of protocol amendments*

- *Concept of protocol exception, deviation and violation*

7.2 Introduction

Every clinical trial (research) starts with the development of a clinical protocol. A protocol is a document which describes how a clinical trial will be conducted. A protocol states clearly the research question and the steps involved in answering that research question. It also ensures the safety of the trial subjects and integrity of the data collected.

7.3 Protocol - Definition

A Clinical Trial Protocol is a document that describes the objective(s), design, methodology, statistical considerations, and the organization of a Clinical Trial.

7.4 Protocol approval

Once the planning stage is completed in a clinical trial, the plan should be documented and this documented plan is known as "research protocol" (plan of trial/study). This protocol needs to be submitted to IRB/IEC for approval. Ethics committee review the submitted documents and check minutely all the details provided in the document. They ensure that the data submitted is sufficient to satisfy the regulatory requirements. With the approval of the study protocol, the trial can be started (refer to the **Fig – Protocol approval**).

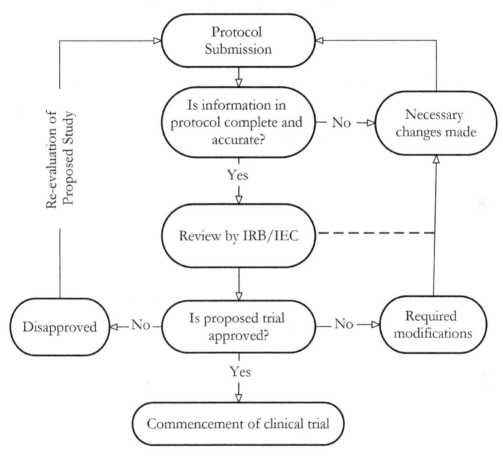

Fig: Protocol approval

7.5 Key elements of the research protocol

A research protocol precisely explains the entire plan for the execution of the trial (refer to the **Fig – Key elements of Protocol**).

7.6 Contents of Research Protocol

According to the ICH Good Clinical Practice guidelines, the contents of a trial protocol should generally include the topics mentioned in the **Fig – Content of protocol**.

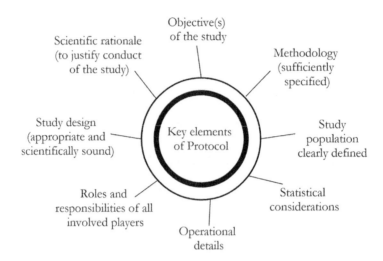

Fig: Key elements of Protocol

* Title page (General Information)	* Assessment of efficacy	* Ethics
* Background information	* Assessment of safety	* Data handling and Record keeping
* Trial objective and purpose	* References	* Financing and Insurance
* Trial design	* Statistics	* Publication policy
* Selection and withdrawal of Subjects	* Direct access to Source data/document	* Adverse events
* Treatment of subjects	* Quality control and Quality assurance	* Supplements/ Appendices

Fig: Content of Protocol

7.7 Need for research protocol

Every research study should have a protocol as the protocol explains the guidelines for conducting the trial. It describes each of the element of the trial and it also guides on how it should be carried out. **Fig – Need for research protocol** explains, why the research protocol is required in a research study.

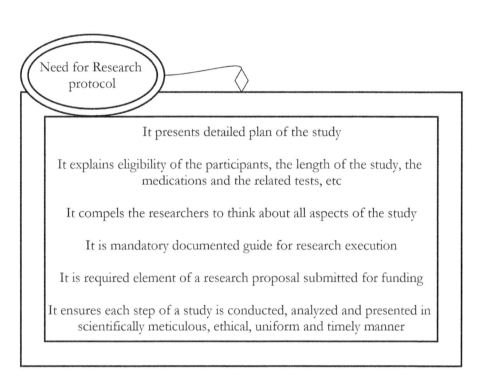

7.8 Importance of Protocol

The study protocol ensures that the required elements of the study has been communicated appropriately and adequately to the investigators, IRB, and regulatory agencies. Thus, the research protocol is an essential part of a research project (refer to the **Fig – Importance of Protocol**).

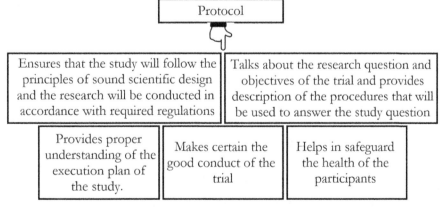

Fig: Importance of Protocol

7.9 Users of Trial/Study Protocol

Protocol is a required document to conduct the trial in a systematic manner. All the players (refer to the **Fig – Users of Study Protocol**) of a trial refer to protocol in order to understand their respective roles in the trial.

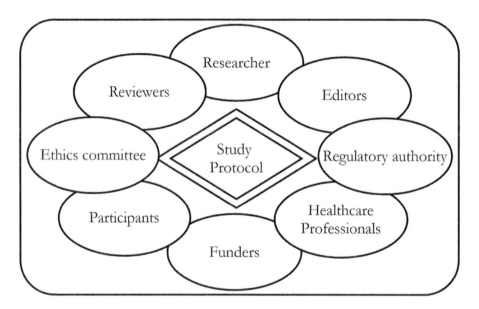

Fig: Users of Study Protocol

7.10 Preparation of Protocol

Protocol depicts the exact plan of study/trial and hence, it should be prepared very carefully by putting in sufficient time and by obtaining inputs from various experts. Protocol is unique and specific for each study and that is the reason due to which the standardized protocol is impossible to come up with for all studies. However, there are certain common sections and informational content found in all the protocols. These common elements can be reused for other protocols but it does not restrict the design of protocol for various studies.

The Clinical Trial Protocol is mostly prepared by the sponsoring company with an input from the Principal Investigator (PI) and the regulatory agencies. But ultimately, the clinical trials are considered sponsored projects and are reviewed and approved as such.

Process of writing Protocol

During the process of development of protocol, it is beneficial for the writer of protocol to discuss with colleagues and experts so that the further refinement of the protocol can be achieved. Precise and concise drafting of a research protocol will increase the chance of getting valid and reliable outcome at the end of the study (refer to the **Fig – Process of writing protocol**). Once the protocol is developed and approved and the study has begun, there should not be any alteration in the approved protocol during the progression of the study/trial. Violations of the protocol can discredit the whole study. If minor changes are done during the progress of the study, then the preferred action will be the exclusion of that part of the study from the analysis.

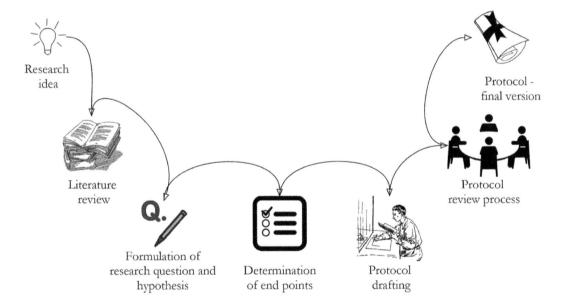

Fig: Process of writing Protocol

The protocol should depict the rationale behind the study, its objective, the methodology used and how the data will be collected and analysed. It should underline, how ethical issues have been considered, and, where suitable, how gender issues are being addressed.

Quality of a protocol can be determined by following criteria

➪ Is it answering the research question(s) sufficiently and thereby achieving the research objective?

➪ Is it workable in the particular research environment for the study?

➪ Is it furnishing adequate information which can be helpful for another researcher to do the research and to elicit comparable inferences?

7.11 Protocol amendment

Protocol amendment is defined as a revision, a change, or an addition (addendum) to an approved research protocol. The IRB reviews and approves all amendments (i.e., revisions, modifications, or addenda) to an IRB approved research protocol. Amendment in protocol during progress of the study can introduce challenges in data analysis and result production. The implementation and communication of amendments can be a costly affair. There are three different types of Protocol amendments (refer to the **Fig: Types of Protocol amendments**).

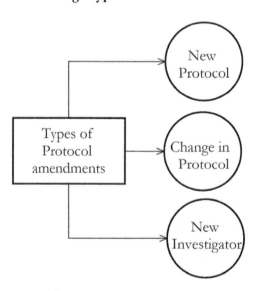

Fig: Types of Protocol amendments

The types of protocol amendment (New protocol, Change in protocol and New Investigator) have been described below:

7.12 New protocol amendment

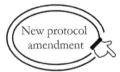

Occurs when sponsors plan to conduct a trial that is not covered by their protocol but which is already contained in their IND (Investigational New Drug) application, then new protocols (new changes) can be submitted to an existing IND

The FDA submission demands a brief description of most clinically significant differences between the new protocol and previously submitted protocol(s).

Submission of copies of IRB approval letters and approved Informed Consent Form documents are required for the FDA to ensure that IRB requirements have been met

7.13 Change in protocol

Change in protocol

Changes to an existing protocol should be submitted to FDA along with a description of the changes.

The amended study can begin once it has been submitted to the FDA for review and the amended study has local IRB approval

These changes in the existing protocol can significantly affect safety of subjects, scope of the investigation, or scientific quality of the study.

Note: A change in protocol intended to eliminate immediate hazards to human subjects may be implemented immediately, provided that FDA is subsequently notified by protocol amendment and the reviewing IRB is also notified.

Examples of protocol changes

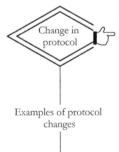

Any increase in drug dosage or duration of exposure to drug

Any significant increase in the planned number of subjects enrolled

Addition of new test procedures or elimination of test procedures

7.14 New investigator

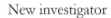

New investigator

A sponsor of an IND application is expected to submit a protocol amendment when a new investigator is added to carry out a previously submitted protocol.

The amendment should include the investigator's name, the qualifications to conduct the investigation, and any reference to the previously submitted protocol, if relevant.

FDA should be notified within 30 days of the investigator being added.

7.15 Protocol Exceptions, Deviations and Violations

- Protocol Exceptions, Deviations and Violations occurs when there is an inconsistency in the research study due to difference between the IRB approved protocol and the actual execution within the research study (these differences are due to some introduced changes in a proposed study)

- These changes in an approved study must be reviewed and approved by IRB before implementing the changes (exception- when necessary to eliminate apparent immediate hazards to the subject in a research study)

- Protocol violation/deviation turns into noncompliance if it is severe/frequent and this may call for a "For-cause audit" of the study

- Immediate reporting to IRB is a must when violation/deviation come into knowledge of any research staff

- Protocol modification is required in case of frequent requests for protocol exceptions

- Protocol Exception, Protocol Deviation and Protocol Violation are explained in the **Fig – Protocol Exceptions, Fig – Protocol Deviation and Fig – Protocol Violation** respectively.

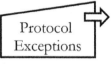 These are intentional deviations from the approved protocol. It is the responsibility of the Investigator to request permission from the IRB for planned exceptions to the approved protocol unless the change is considered necessary to eliminate an obvious immediate hazard.

Example - accommodation of a study subject who moves out of the area for the remainder of his/her participation in the research

Fig: Protocol Exceptions

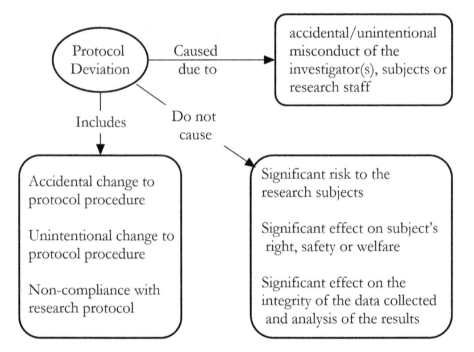

Example of protocol deviation

Rescheduled study visit - performing a planned procedure on a different timetable than previously specified in the research protocol because of an unexpected interference such as a subject's vacation

Fig: Protocol Deviation

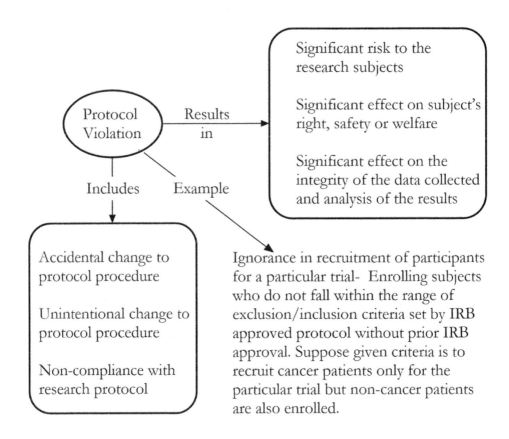

Fig: Protocol Violation

Chapter 8

INFORMED CONSENT

8.1 Learnings from the chapter

- *Introduction to Informed Consent with its purpose, importance and types*
- *Guiding principles and elements of informed consent*
- *Details about segments, language, classification and revision of informed consent form*
- *Informed consent process with its documentation details*
- *Concept of re-consenting and therapeutic misconception*
- *Exceptions to informed consent rule*

8.2 Introduction

Every year, a number of clinical trials are conducted in the field of healthcare and needless to say these trials need a good number of volunteers who are required to participate and allow the testing of new treatment in their body. Prior to the agreement to participate in a trial, the volunteers must understand what they are going to do in a trial process. They must converse with concerned people in detail about each and every aspect of the trial and then they should decide whether to participate in the trial or not. Here comes the concept of Informed Consent (IC).

8.3 Definition of Informed Consent

"An informed consent is a process by which a subject voluntarily confirms his or her willingness to participate in a particular trial, after having been informed of all aspects of the trial that are relevant to the subject's decision to participate. Informed consent is documented by means of a written, signed and dated informed consent form (ICF)."

Informed consent process is all about the protection and respect for the research subjects. Informed consent is a precondition for the volunteer's participation in the trial. It must be done before enrolling any participant in any type of trial which involves human subject. The aim of the informed consent process is to provide sufficient information to the interested volunteers which enables them to make conscious decision on whether to participate or not to participate in a trial/study or to continue participation in the trial/study.

8.4 Purpose of Informed Consent

Volunteers, who are interested to participate in a trial must be made aware of the fact that the trials are different from the standard medical practices. Before starting any research, the participants must be informed about all the aspects of the trial. Informed consent serves this purpose (refer to the **Fig – Purpose of Informed consent**).

Informed Consent helps in

Maintaining and respecting subject's will

Explaining individual's rights of participation in the trial

Keeping informed the human subjects about aim, procedure, risk, benefits and other various aspects of the trial

Voluntarily decision making about participation in the trial

Fig: Purpose of Informed Consent

8.5 Importance of Informed Consent

Informed consent is a person's voluntary consent to participate in a trial after being aware of all relevant aspects of the trial. The important roles of the Informed Consent in making the interested volunteers aware regarding the various aspects of the trial has been depicted in the **Fig – Importance of Informed Consent**.

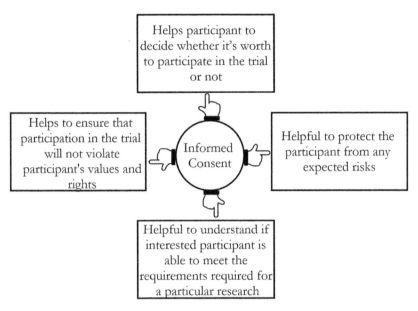

Fig: Importance of Informed Consent

Some important terms

Legally Authorized Representatives (LAR) - An individual or a judicial or any other body authorized under applicable law to give consent on behalf of a prospective subject to the subject's participation in the procedure(s) involved in the research.

Capacity – A onetime clinical judgment of a client's ability to give informed consent i.e., decision made by a healthcare professional regarding a patient's ability to make a specific decision at a specific time.

Competence – The ability to understand legal rights and responsibilities and the possession of authority to make legal decisions.

Impartial Witness - Impartial Witness is "a person, (a) who is independent of the trial, (b) who cannot be unfairly influenced by people involved with the trial, (c) who attends the informed consent process if the subject or the subject's legally acceptable representative cannot read, and (d) who reads the informed consent form and any other written information supplied to the subject."

All prospective subjects must have the capacity and competence to provide legally effective informed consent for participation in a particular trial. Individuals who do not have such ability (i.e. capacity and competence) can only be enrolled in research through consent of their legally authorized representative (LAR).

8.6 Guiding principles of Informed Consent process

ICF is an essential document of a clinical trial and it is a compulsory part of a protocol. It must contain all elements required by the regulations (refer to the **Fig – Sources of principles of Informed Consent**).

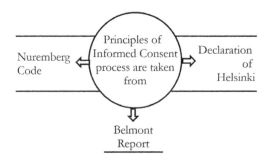

Fig: Sources of principles of Informed Consent

The informed consent Form (ICF) must be approved by an institutional review board (IRB)/ independent ethics committee (IEC).

8.7 Elements of Informed consent

According to the regulations, Informed consent document contains basic and additional elements (refer to the **Fig-Elements of Informed Consent**).

8.8 Basic elements of Informed Consent (In detail)

• Purposes - This is a statement which indicates that the study involves research, an explanation of the purposes of the research, the expected duration of the subject's participation, a description of the procedures to be followed, identification of procedures which are experimental.

• Risks - This is a description of any reasonably foreseeable risks or discomforts which may come to the subject.

• Benefits - This is a description of any benefits to the subject or to others which may reasonably be expected from the research.

• Alternatives treatments - This is a disclosure of appropriate alternative procedures or the courses of treatment, if any, that might be advantageous to the subject.

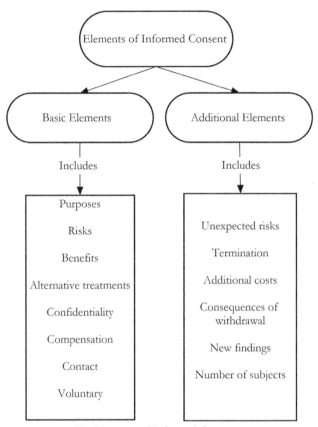

Fig: Elements of Informed Consent

- Confidentiality - This is a statement describing the extent, if any, to which the confidentiality of records identifying the subject will be maintained.

- Compensation - For research involving more than minimal risk, an explanation as to whether any compensation and/or any medical treatments are available, if injury occurs and, if so, what they consist of, or from where any further information may be obtained.

- Contact - This is an explanation of whom to contact for answers to pertinent questions about the research and research subject's rights and, whom to contact in the event of a research-related injury to the subject.

- Voluntary - This is a statement which means that participation is voluntary. Refusal to participate will involve no penalty or loss of benefits which the subject is otherwise entitled to, and the subject may discontinue participation at any time without facing any penalty or loss of benefits, which the subject is otherwise entitled to.

8.9 Additional elements of informed consent (in detail)

- Unexpected risks - This is a statement that a particular treatment or a procedure may involve risks to the subject (or to the embryo or foetus, in case the subject is or may become pregnant), which are currently unforeseeable.

- Termination - This refers to anticipated circumstances under which the subject's participation may be terminated by the investigator, without regard to the subject's consent.

- Additional costs - This refers to any additional costs to the subject that may result from participation in the research.

- Consequences of withdrawal - This refers to the consequences of a subject's decision to withdraw from the research and the procedures for orderly termination of participation by the subject.

- New findings - This is a statement that the significant new findings developed during the research, which may relate to the subject's willingness to continue participation, will be provided to the subject.

- Number of subjects - This refers to the approximate number of subjects involved in the study.

8.10 Segments of Informed Consent Form (ICF)

Informed consent form (ICF) consist of two segments i.e. Patient information sheet and Consent certificate (refer to the **Fig – Segments of ICF**).

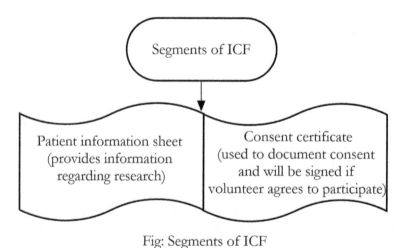

Fig: Segments of ICF

8.11 Language of Informed Consent Form (ICF)

ICF is not only a form. It is also a process which provides the necessary information regarding a trial to the interested volunteers. It must be written in a language that can be easily understood by the volunteers and it must minimize the possibility of coercion or undue influence (refer to the **Fig – Language of an ICF**).

Clearly written and understandable to the volunteers
Use of easy language and small words
For a non-English speaking participant, consent document should be translated in participant's preferred language and this translated document should be approved by IRB
Scientific, technical, and medical terms must be explained properly
The language must be non-technical to the extent possible
Recommended reading level of the informed consent should be the sixth or eighth grade reading level
In case of minor (as a participant) in a study, related recruitment materials must reflect the reading level of minors
It must avoid the reflection of any type of insistence or undue influence on the participant

Fig: Language of an ICF

8.12 Classification of Informed Consent Form

Informed Consent Forms can be classified as Written consent and Short form written consent (refer to the **Fig- Classification of Informed Consent Form**).

Exculpatory language should be excluded in oral or written informed consent. The difference between above two is that written consent form presents everything in written while short form presents orally as well.

8.13 Informed Consent - Designing

Informed consent form (final version) should be designed appropriately to serve the right purpose and this assurance comes from combined effort of different players in a clinical trial (refer to the **Fig- Final drafting of Informed consent form**).

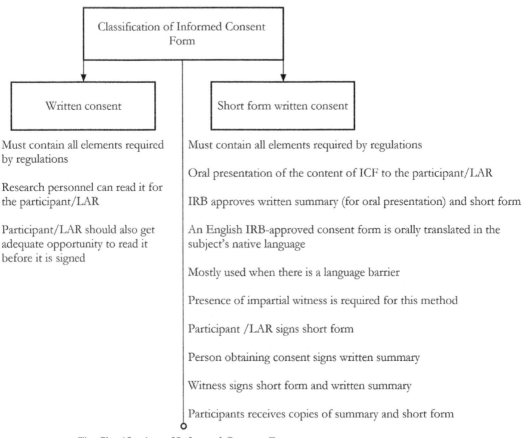

Fig: Classification of Informed Consent Form

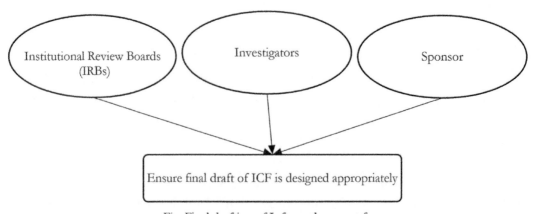

Fig: Final drafting of Informed consent form

8.14 Informed Consent Process

Informed consent is an ongoing process which involves communication and mutual understanding between the researcher and the participant. Hence, informed consent process is a kind of agreement between researcher and subject, which should be signed once the participant has understood the trial and its implications thoroughly and he/she is ready to participate in the trial voluntarily.

Informed consent process should take place in a safe, private, quiet and comfortable place. Generally principal investigator, sub-investigator or IRB approved personnel interview the prospective participants. Typically, informed consent has to be signed before the start of the trial. The informed consent process involves following steps (refer to the **Fig – Informed consent process**).

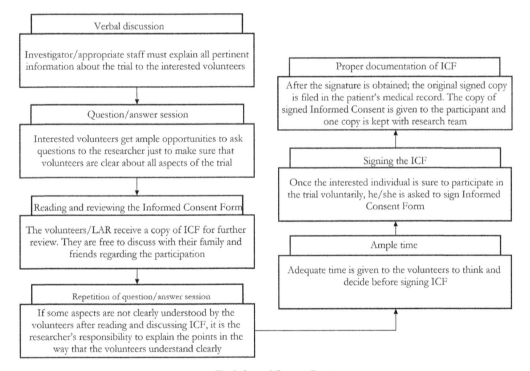

Fig: Informed Consent Process

8.15 Documentation of Informed Consent Form

Documentation of informed consent is a crucial step in a trial. It reflects that the informed consent process has been followed properly. The person signing the ICF must be qualified enough to attest to the fact that the subject has provided legally effective informed consent. However, many research personnel are involved in this process, but the Principal Investigator is ultimately responsible for the informed consent process. In the absence of Principal investigator, a sub-investigator with appropriate qualification and expertise can play the same role.

Depending upon the situation, ICF must be signed by the subject/subject's LAR/parents in case of child participant (refer to the **Fig-Signing of ICF**).

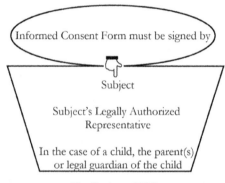

Fig: Signing of ICF

The signing of ICF by the research personnel before obtaining the signature of the subject is not an acceptable practice. Normally, the signing procedure should take place in the presence of both the parties (research personnel and participant).

8.16 Revision of Informed Consent Form

There can be chances of revisions in the research ICF during the trial process (refer to the **Fig-Revision of ICF**). The revised informed consent document must be approved by IRB/IEC prior to the same being put in use.

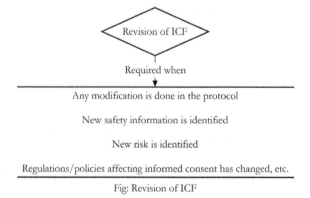

Fig: Revision of ICF

8.17 Re-consenting

Participants must be well informed about any new information or any new change in a trial that may impact the participant's willingness to take part in the research. Therefore, it is the responsibility of the principal investigator to make sure that the written documentation of the re-consent is obtained at various intervals of the trial process. The informed consent process with the new information needs to be repeated with every clinical trial participant. The participant is then required to sign the revised form. The documentation of signed ICF (revised) should be done properly.

8.18 Types of Informed Consent

There are different kinds of Informed Consent which are available for the purpose of a research (refer to the **Fig – Types of Informed Consent**).

Consent An adult subject above 18 years (having capacity and competence) can give consent for participation in a research study	Assent Assent is a child's (age 7-17 years) affirmative agreement to participate in a research	Short Form Generally used when there is a language barrier and an English IRB approved consent is orally presented to the participants in their native language
Information/Fact Sheet It is used in certain circumstances such as when signed consent is not required by the regulations	Verbal The participant verbally reads and verbally agrees to participate in a research (Verbal consent contains all elements of written consent)	Parental Permission When children/minors are involved in research, the parent/guardian must sign a parental permission consent document
Waiver of Documentation of Informed Consent Often used in minimal risk research involving the administration of online or mailed surveys, telephone interviews, or when anonymous sensitive information is collected and participants do not want any written link for participation to the research.	Waiver of Elements of Informed Consent It is obtained from the IRB for some research categories, which are not possible to conduct without an alteration to the required elements	

Fig: Types of Informed Consent

8.19 Therapeutic misconception

Consider an instance like this one: - A patient goes to a physician for routine medical care; the physician discusses with patient about research study treatment and other aspects; the patient misinterprets the information and enrolls in the study assuming he is taking normal medical treatment. Hence, it the responsibility of the physician to make it very clear to the patient, that he will be enrolled for a trial treatment not routine treatment.

8.20 Vulnerable population - Consent

Persons who are relatively or completely incapable of protecting their own interests are termed as vulnerable population (refer to the **Fig – Vulnerable population**).

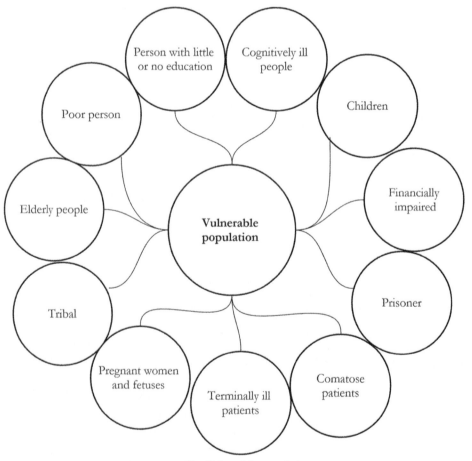

Fig: Vulnerable population

During the process of taking consent from vulnerable population, the researcher and the ethics committee need to ensure that the participants are not being exploited and their safety and dignity is being maintained in every situation. The consent of a child will be required in addition to that of the parent. Researcher should make sure that they present the whole matter in such a way that a child can understand the clauses completely. A research is justified only if the research is responsive to the health needs and priorities of the vulnerable population and that the research stands to benefit from the results of the research.

8.21 Research involving children

Clinical research which involves children as participants, must be handled with proper care. This kind of research may need both the Consent and the Assent. Few points related to research in children are mentioned in the **Fig – Research involving Children**.

IAF (Informed Assent Form) is used for obtaining the consent of children wherein this form should be written in the language which is appropriate to the age group of the children. This form is signed in addition to ICF (parental consent).

Prior to taking consent and assent with the intent to involve children in research, it is a must to explain that comparable research cannot be done with adults to the same effect and scientific impact.

Age for informed assent varies but it is good for researcher to consider taking the assent for 7 years and above age group.

Children who are able to understand the research aspects, should get sufficient opportunity to be informed about all the aspects and also to question regarding research.

They should also be provided an opportunity to express their willingness on whether to participate or not to participate. Assent denied by child should be taken seriously.

Fig: Research involving children

8.22 Exceptions to the informed consent rule

Under certain circumstances, there are some exceptions to the informed consent rule (refer to the **Fig – Informed consent rule – Exceptions**).

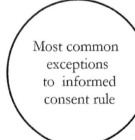 An emergency in which medical care is needed immediately to prevent serious or irreversible harm

Incompetence in which someone is unable to give permission (or to refuse permission) for testing or treatment

Fig: Informed consent rule - Exceptions

Informed consent process starts before the start of the study and it gets over once study is completed and final reports are published.

Chapter 9

HUMAN PARTICIPATION IN CLINICAL TRIAL (RESEARCH)

9.1 Learnings from the chapter

- *Details about human participation in a clinical trial which includes selection, recruitment and retention of human subjects*

- *Types of volunteers in a clinical trial*

- *Various aspects of recruitment process such as recruitment strategies, recruitment methods, recruitment difficulties, etc.*

- *Details about selection of potential candidates, enrolment planning, retention strategies and other factors related to subject's participation*

- *Compensation to human subjects in a clinical trial*

- *Ethical concerns in recruitment process and compliance to a trial*

9.2 Introduction

Clinical research uses volunteers (human subjects) to scientifically prove the safety and efficacy of an experimental treatment for further use in the general population. Clinical research cannot run without human volunteers. Hence, the adequate recruitment of volunteers and their retention is one of the important factors for the success of long run trials.

9.3 Types of Volunteers in Clinical Trial

Volunteers can be of two types i.e., healthy volunteers and patient volunteers (refer to the **Fig- Types of volunteers in a clinical trial**).

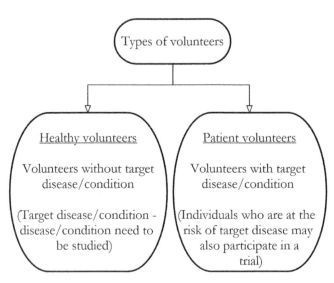

Fig: Types of volunteers in a clinical trial

9.4 Participation of human beings in a trial

Participation of human beings (as study/trial subjects) in a clinical trial depends on three important elements i.e. selection, recruitment and retention (refer to the **Fig- Key elements of volunteer's participation in clinical trial**).

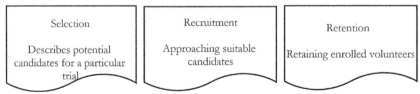

Fig: Key elements of volunteer's participation in clinical trial

9.5 Factors to be considered prior to the start of recruitment process

Recruitment process (of volunteers for the trial) can be tedious and time consuming. Proper planning can be very helpful in achieving the recruitment targets within the defined timeline. Prior to the enrolment process, the research team must plan and assess their resources, their objectives and actions. Focused work will save money and time in long run and will also help to run the trial smoothly. Few factors which must be considered in advance before starting the recruitment process are mentioned in the **Fig-Factors to be considered prior to start of recruitment process**.

Proper planning	Budgeting	Recruitment metrics
During designing protocol, it is good to plan for recruitment process also such as where the recruitment will take place, what will be the mode of recruitment, timeline for recruitment process, who will be responsible for recruitment process, etc	Financial planning helps to estimate and manage the whole recruitment process smoothly otherwise there can be possibility of inadequate recruitment of volunteers due to ill management of finances which may lead to invalid results	Evaluation of effectiveness of recruitment process through recruitment metrics helps to understand the gaps in planned strategies which also unfolds the pros and cons of using different recruitment methods. Thus, metrics helps in taking important measures to achieve the target in set timeline

Monitoring	Training
It is good to keep an eye on every little and large step for successful completion of trial	Proper training of the research staff ensures proper conduct of trial steps

Fig: Factors to be considered prior to start of recruitment process

9.6 Enrolment planning

Recruitment process starts with identification of target audience. It is always good to start contacting the potential volunteers who are well qualified and easy to contact. It saves a lot of time (as in convincing and contacting). Few other tips related to proper planning of enrolment are listed in the **Fig – Enrolment planning.**

Internal recruitment should be preferred (Internal recruitment refers to enrolment of patient who are familiar with research site and their research plan)

Options that cost less to the research team should be opted first. Example- healthcare provider referrals, social networking, etc.

Tips for successful enrolment planning

Correct and fair estimation of the research site feasibility for enrolment of participants is a great help for the research team to plan the overall process

Emails, phone calls, advertisement, social media, internal database are other options that are of help in completing the enrolment process

Fig: Enrolment planning

9.7 Selection of potential participant

Clinical research involves volunteers (human subjects) not with the intent to directly benefit them (volunteers) from the trial, but to develop a new knowledge and an understanding about the medical field. Hence, a person who is interested to participate in a trial must understand the difference between the routine medical treatment and the clinical trial. Individuals who want to participate in a trial need to understand the potential benefits and the risks of participation in a clinical trial.

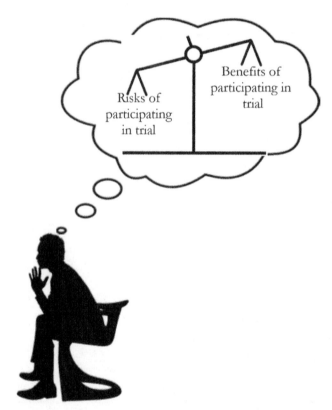

Fig: Volunteer thinking to participate in a clinical trial

9.8 Eligibility criteria and selection process

Interested candidates must fulfil the eligibility criteria set by the particular trial. Individuals who do not qualify these criteria, cannot participate in that particular trial. These criteria vary from trial to trial.

Eligibility criteria helps to extract the potential participants. Each clinical trial follows specific guidelines regarding the selection of potential participants. Eligibility criteria consist of two fragments i.e. exclusion criteria and inclusion criteria [refer to the **Fig-Eligibility criteria (with impacting factors)**].

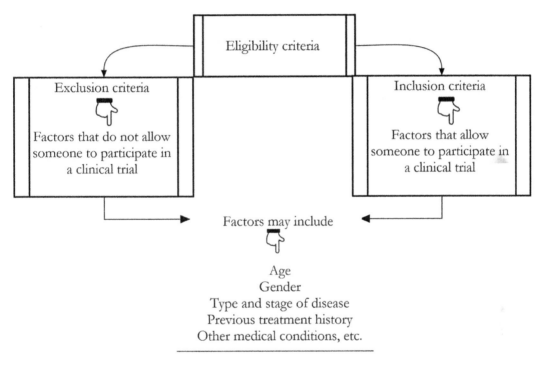

Fig: Eligibility criteria (with impacting factors)

The main benefit of eligibility criteria is that these criteria avoid rejection or selection of people on personal basis (refer to the **Fig – Importance of Eligibility Criteria**). These criteria describe the characteristics that must be minimally shared by all the participants. Enrolling participants with similar characteristics ensure that the result obtained at the end of the trial is due to investigational factor and not due to other factors.

9.9 Factors which motivate the volunteers to participate in a trial

There are many reasons (refer to the **Fig – Factors which motivate volunteers to participate in a trial**) which can motivate the volunteers to participate or to continue with their participation in a trial.

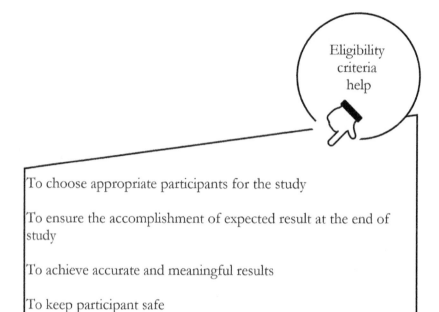

To choose appropriate participants for the study

To ensure the accomplishment of expected result at the end of study

To achieve accurate and meaningful results

To keep participant safe

Fig: Importance of Eligibility Criteria

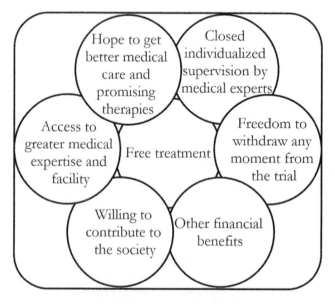

Fig: Factors which motivate volunteers to
participate in a trial

9.10 Factors which de-motivate the volunteers to participate in a trial

There are many reasons (refer to the **Fig – Factors which de-motivate volunteers to participate or to continue their participation in a trial**) which can de-motivate the volunteers with respect to their participation or with respect to their continued participation in a trial.

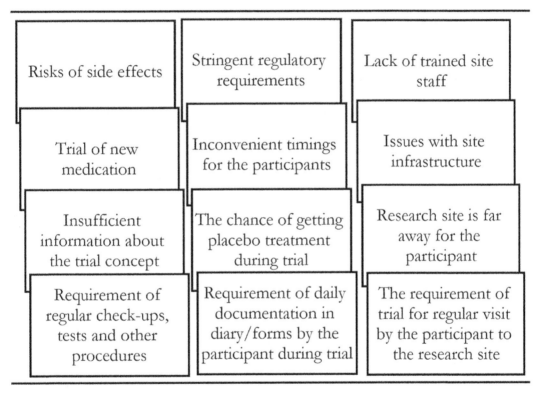

Fig: Factors which de-motivate volunteers to participate or to continue their participation in a trial

9.11 Recruitment strategies

There are different recruitment strategies that can be used for different trials (depending upon the requirement of the trial). Selection of correct strategy helps in adequate enrolment of volunteers for the trial process. Recruitment strategies vary from trial to trial depending on the research question, context of research, site of investigation, etc. Few examples of recruitment strategies are listed in **Fig – Examples of recruitment strategy**.

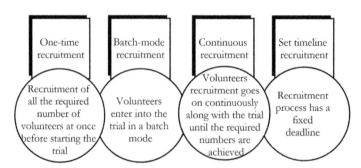

Fig: Examples of recruitment strategy

9.12 Recruitment Process

Recruitment process of interested volunteers in a clinical trial follows steps depicted in the **Fig – Steps of recruitment process.**

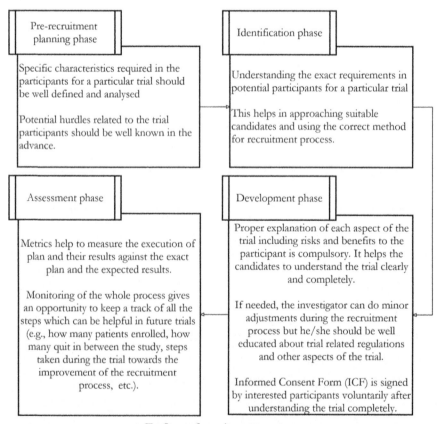

Fig: Steps of recruitment process

9.13 Recruitment methods

There are various methods through which the potential participants can be approached to get them into the trial. Few examples are mentioned in the **Fig- Recruitment methods**.

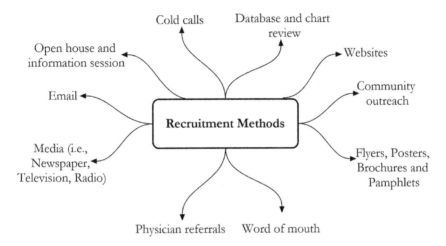

Fig: Recruitment methods

9.14 Different factors and recruitment rate

Recruitment rate depends on multiple factors. Some of the factors are listed in the **Fig – Factors affecting recruitment rate**.

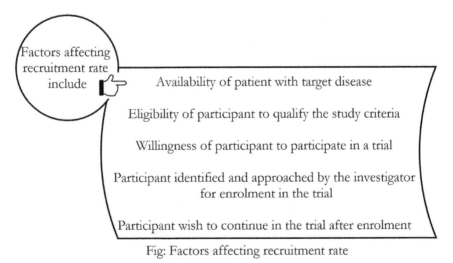

Fig: Factors affecting recruitment rate

9.15 Difficulties in the recruitment process

Even though the appropriate recruitment methods can enhance the number of enrolments, there are reasons which can create obstacles in the recruitment process. Some of those reasons are listed in the **Fig – Difficulties in recruitment process**.

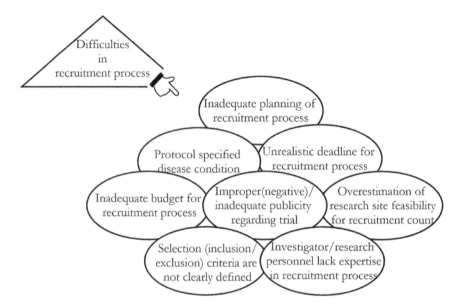

Fig: Difficulties in recruitment process

9.16 Recruitment success tips

The presence of an active investigator and other research staff in a trial is the primary requirement for the success of a recruitment process in a trial. Apart from this, some other important tips which can be helpful in making a recruitment process successful are mentioned in **Fig – Tips for recruitment success**.

9.17 Retention of the participants

To maintain the validity of the data during the trial, it is required to retain the recruited subjects. In some cases, the subjects show disinterest in further participation because they may have received some inaccurate information or they may be having some personal problems. Hence, once the participants are enrolled in the trial, it is the responsibility of the site staff to keep the participant motivated and positive regarding the participation in the trial. Participants should be treated well and they should feel comfortable during the trial. They should be well

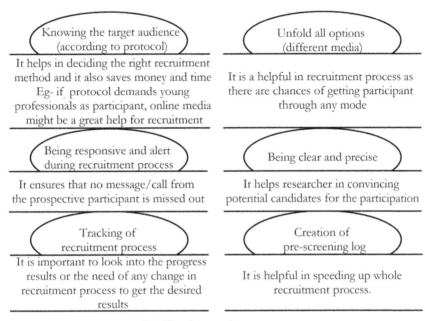

Fig: Tips for recruitment success

informed about all the trial activities. These small efforts from the research team can retain the participant till the end in most of the cases.

However, sometimes despite of all positive environments, the participant wishes to withdraw from the study. In some cases, the investigator may discontinue the subject from participation in the trial. Sometimes, the trial is terminated in between by sponsor due to some reason such as safety concern, business reasons, etc.

9.18 Reasons for the dropout of the subject from the trial

Interested participants take part in the trial, but sometimes they drop the idea of continuing their participation in the trial. Some common reasons of the withdrawing of the subject from the trial can be referred in the **Fig – Various reasons for subject's dropout from the trial.**

9.19 Reasons behind the investigator expecting the subject to pull out from the trial

Apart from the subject of the trial, sometimes the investigator also takes the decision to remove the subject from the trial because of some issues (refer to the **Fig- Reasons behind investigator expecting the subject to discontinue from the trial**) which can impact the outcome of trial.

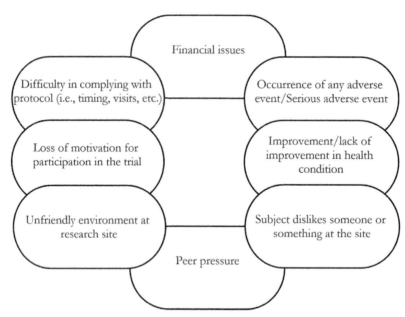

Fig: Various reasons for subject's dropout from the trial

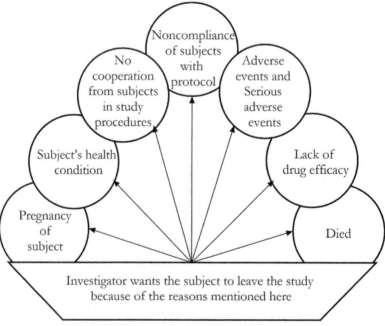

Fig: Reasons behind investigator expecting the subject to
discontinue from the trial

9.20 Retention strategies to avoid dropouts

There are various ways through which study subjects can be retained in the trial. Some of those ways are listed in the **Fig – Retention strategies.**

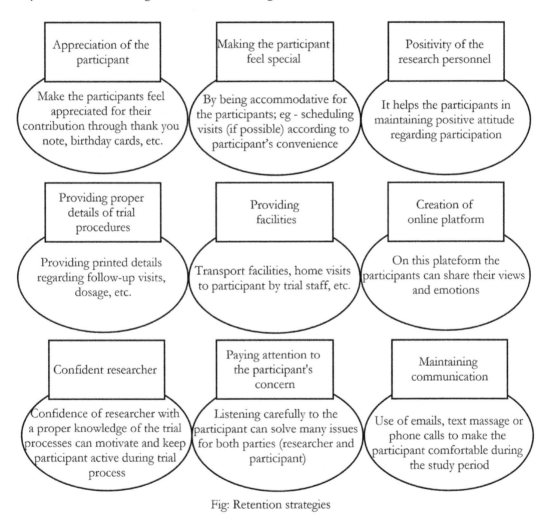

Fig: Retention strategies

9.21 Compensation to the subjects

Subjects are compensated for participating in a trial and these compensations must be approved by IRB in advance. Prior to the approval of compensation, IRB ensures that it does not cause any coerciveness and undue influence on subject's decision regarding the participation in a trial.

The amount of compensation varies from trial to trial. Compensation usually includes costs to the subjects due to participation in the trial such as transport, lunch, childcare, etc. Compensation should not be so large that it only becomes the reason for participation.

However, some trials do not offer compensation which is also acceptable.

9.22 Compliance to trial

The main objective of a clinical trial is to assess safety and efficacy of a new medical product/ treatment. Hence, it is necessary for all players in clinical trial to be compliant with protocol because any noncompliance may lead to invalid results. Noncompliance can lead to following conclusions (refer to the **Fig – Impact of non-compliance in a clinical trial**) which can be harmful for general public.

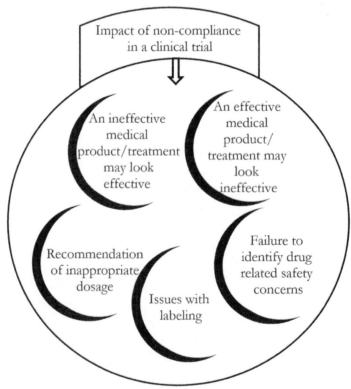

Fig: Impact of non-compliance in a clinical trial

In case of the subject, poor compliance or noncompliance can be due to many reasons (refer to the **Fig – Reason's for subject's poor compliance/non-compliance in a clinical trial**).

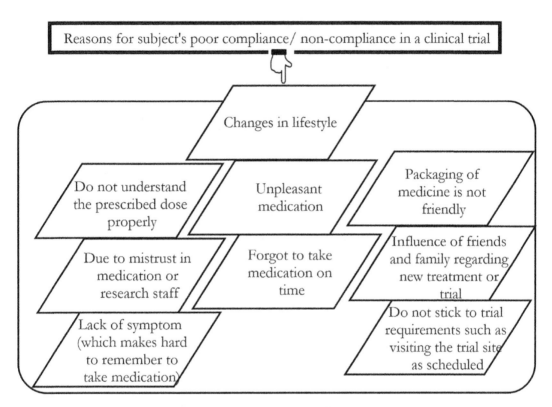

Fig: Reasons for subject's poor compliance/noncompliance in a clinical trial

To achieve a valid outcome at the end of the study, the investigator and the clinical research coordinator (CRC) should ensure that the subjects are compliant to the protocol (refer to the **Fig – Role of Investigator and CRC in maintaining compliance in a trial**). The investigator and CRC must explain properly to the subjects regarding the importance of compliance in a study. They should give the details to the subjects stating on how being irresponsible regarding procedures can impact the whole study result negatively and ultimately the whole general population.

9.23 Ethical concerns in recruitment process

Recruitment processes must maintain the social value of the research. These should minimize risk and enhance the benefits to the enrolled subjects. These processes should also take care of enhancement of the scientific validity. Some of the important points relevant from the ethical perspective are discussed in the **Fig – Ethical concern in recruitment process**.

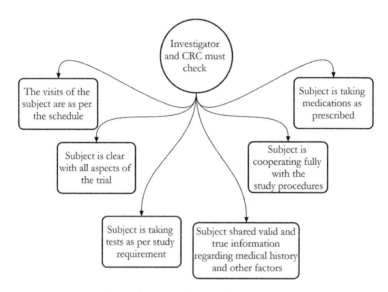

Fig: Role of Investigator and CRC in maintaining compliance in a trial

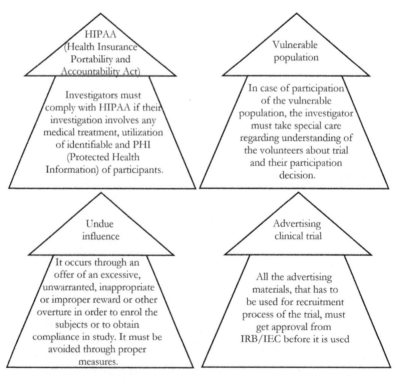

Fig: Ethical concern in recruitment process

Chapter 10

RANDOMIZATION AND BLINDING

10.1 Learnings from the chapter

- *Types of errors (random and systematic)*
- *Definition of Bias and details about its different types*
- *Concept of Randomization and different types of randomization*
- *Description of Blinding and its different types*
- *Unblinding*

10.2 Introduction

An error can be defined as the difference between the true value of a measurement and the recorded value of a measurement. Error in clinical study is common to happen and can occur due to many reasons. Errors in trial result in wrong conclusions at the end of a trial and hence, it should be resolved with proper methods.

10.3 Types of Errors

Error can be of two types i.e., random or systematic (refer to the **Fig – Types of Error with their features**).

10.4 Bias

Bias is the tendency to have an opinion, or a view, that is often dominant on assessment of any situation or on drawing any conclusion without considering the real evidence and other relevant information. It is an inclination or preference that influences judgment from being balanced or even-handed.

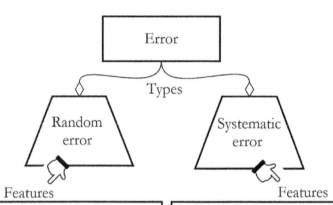

FIg: Types of error with their features

Bias in clinical research can be described as a "systematic distortion/error of the estimated intervention effect away from the truth, that can result in false treatment effect estimates. It can be caused by insufficiencies in the design, conduct or analysis of a trial which leads to inaccurate results. Hence, bias is considered as the most unwanted element in a trial (refer to the **Fig – Occurrence of bias in a clinical trial**). Randomized Controlled Trial (RCT) is known to have potential to reduce/eliminate bias to the maximum.

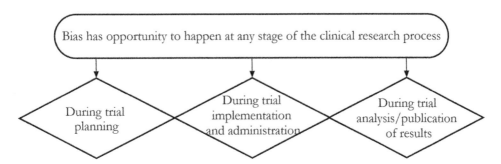

Fig: Occurence of bias in a clinical trial

10.5 Types of Bias

There are a number of types of bias described in clinical research. Major types are listed in the **Fig – Different types of Bias**.

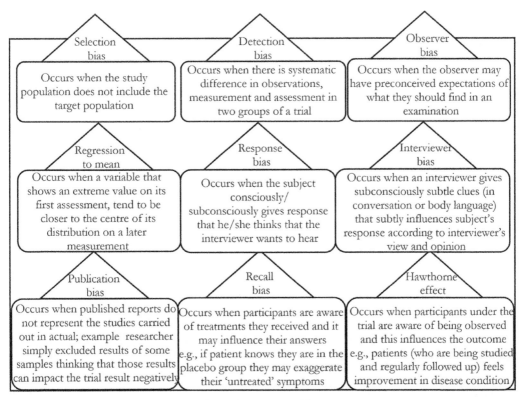

Fig: Different types of Bias

10.6 Steps taken to avoid errors in clinical trial

Randomization and Blinding are the steps taken to avoid errors in a clinical trial. Randomization helps to reduce/eliminate selection bias and confounding factors in a trial while blinding reduces the chances of bias which can be introduced after the allocation of the intervention.

10.7 Randomization –concept in simple terms

During the selection of a football team in a school, there are 7 equally potential candidates who can be selected for the role of goalkeeper. The football coach of the school plans a fair selection process for the goalkeeper slot and he decides to go with the lottery system. He writes the names of the 7 potential candidates on individual chits and put them all in a box. Then he asks the team captain to randomly pick just one chit from the box. The captain picked up 1 chit and thus the 1 goalkeeper got selected out of 7 equally potential candidates. This method eliminated chances of being bias. This process is called randomization.

10.8 Advantages of Randomization in clinical trial

Randomization refers to the practice of using chance methods (random number tables, flipping a coin, etc.) to assign subjects to treatments. The primary advantages of the implementation of randomization in a trial are listed in the **Fig – Advantages of Randomization in clinical trial**.

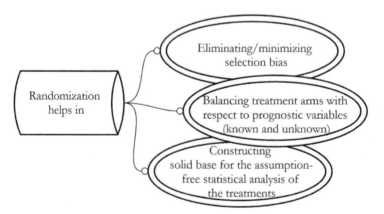

Fig: Advantages of Randomization in clinical trial

10.9 Types of randomization

Randomization plays a very important role in the trial as it ensures that all the participants of a study get an equal chance of being selected into either experimental group or control group. This process leads to uninfluenced (by the investigator or participant) assignment of participants to either intervention. In a research, there are number of ways to do randomization to achieve unbiased and true results. Few such ways are depicted below in the **Fig – Types of Randomization**.

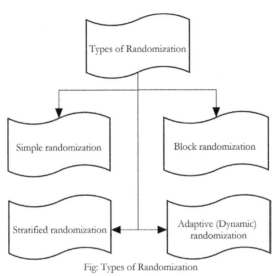

Fig: Types of Randomization

10.10 Simple randomization

It involves random assignment of participants to equally sized treatment groups. Important features of simple randomization are mentioned in the **Fig – Features of Simple randomization**.

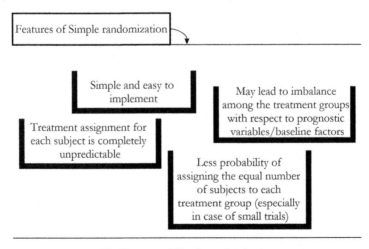

Fig: Features of Simple randomization

Examples of simple randomization

I. Tossing the coin: The sides of a coin would be used to decide the treatment group for the participants. Hence, on tossing the coin, if heads appear, the subject will be assigned to experimental group and if tail appears, the subject would be assigned to the control group (refer to the **Fig – Tossing a coin**).

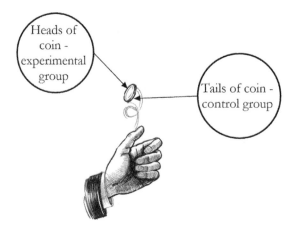

Fig: Tossing a coin

II. Sequence of random numbers from statistical book: e.g., odd number will correspond to the subject getting assigned to the experimental group, whereas even number would lead to the subject getting assigned to the control group.

III. Similarly, Shuffled deck of cards, Throwing of dice, computer generated random numbers are few other examples of simple randomization.

10.11 Block randomization

Block randomization is designed to randomize subjects into groups (block) that results in equal sample sizes. Important features of Block randomization are mentioned in the **Fig – Features of Block randomization**.

Example of Block randomization

Subgroups are created on the basis of gender. Suppose subgroup (block) A has 200 males and subgroup (block) B has 200 females. Now, the treatments (standard and experimental) are assigned randomly within groups. Hence, 100 males out of 200 males receive standard

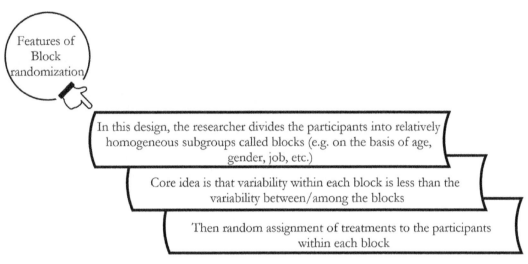

Fig: Features of Block randomization

treatment and rest 100 males receive experimental treatment in subgroup A. Similarly, 100 females are exposed to standard treatment and 100 females are exposed to experimental treatment in subgroup B.

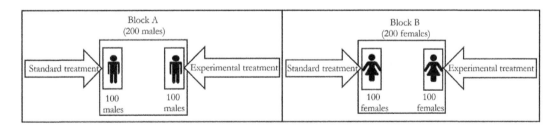

Now, results collected at the end of study will be fair enough as treatments (Experimental and standard) are done equally on both genders and thereby elimination of impact which may occur due to physiological differences factor (due to gender difference).

Gender	Total subject number (in block)	Standard Treatment	Experimental treatment
Male	200	100	100
Female	200	100	100

10.12 Stratified randomization

Stratified randomization is also known as "Stratified Permuted Block Randomization". Stratification means having separate block randomization method for each combination of variables (stratum). In this method, the participants are divided into strata. Strata are constructed on the basis of the baseline characteristics (clinical/prognostic factors) of the participant. Sizes of strata can vary. Then, each stratum is exposed with randomization separately. Important features of Stratified randomization are mentioned in the **Fig – Features of Stratified randomization**.

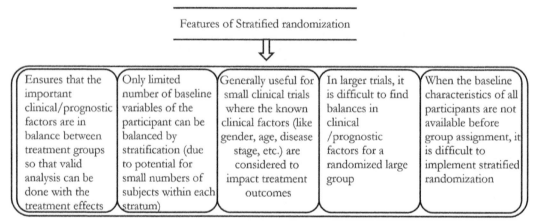

Fig: Features of Stratified randomization

Example of Stratified randomization

Suppose, two prognostic factors are taken into consideration i.e. gender and weight and on the basis of these factors four strata are constructed as follows:

Strata	Standard Treatment	Control treatment
Male - weight<45	13	12
Male - weight>45	40	40
Female - weight <45	12	12
Female - weight>45	39	40

Then, each stratum is exposed to randomization separately. It is advisable to form strata with the most important variables and keep the strata number minimum (as much as possible) as large number of strata can end up with very few participants in each stratum (sometimes, only one participant or even zero participant in each stratum).

10.13 Adaptive (Dynamic) randomization

In this method, the probability of treatment assignment can be adjusted i.e. probability of treatment assignment changes according to the assigned treatments of patients already in the trial. Interim analysis is carried out at several points in time and depending on the circumstances, changes (such as stopping one treatment arm or changing the number of participants in a group) can be made in the trial.

For instance, if the interim analysis demonstrates that a smaller sample size will still provide a valid result at the end of study, then the planned number of participants might be reduced. In the similar way, if analysis demonstrates that increased sample size can help in achieving a valid result within a more acceptable period of time, then the planned number of participants might be increased. Interim analyses and any anticipated changes to a trial should be described and justified in the study protocol. Important features of Adaptive randomization are mentioned in the **Fig – Features of Adaptive randomization**.

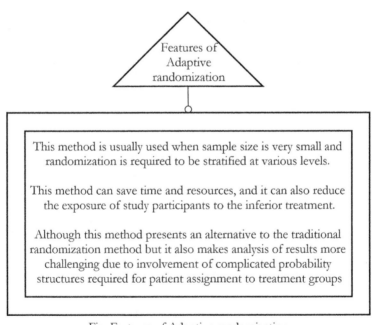

Fig: Features of Adaptive randomization

10.14 Use of different types of randomization in different situations

The factors which can influence the selection of the type of randomization for a particular trial is depicted in the **Fig – Use of different randomization in different situations.**

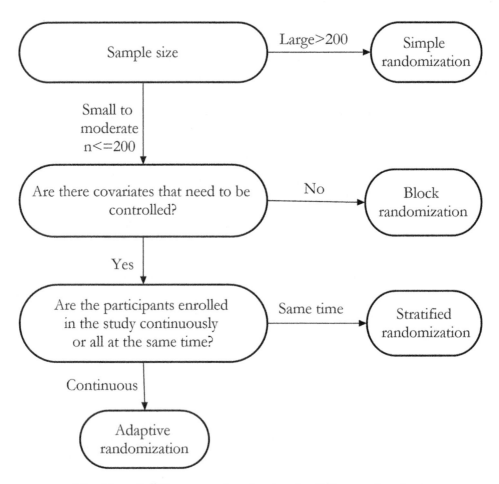

Fig: Use of different randomization in different situation

10.15 Blinding

Blinding is a procedure in which one or more parties in a trial are kept unaware of which treatment arms the participants have been assigned to. Blinding is an important aspect of any trial and it is done in order to avoid and prevent conscious or unconscious bias in the design and execution of a clinical trial.

10.16 Advantages of Blinding in clinical trial

The major advantages of blinding implementation in a trial are described in the **Fig – Advantages of Blinding in clinical trial.**

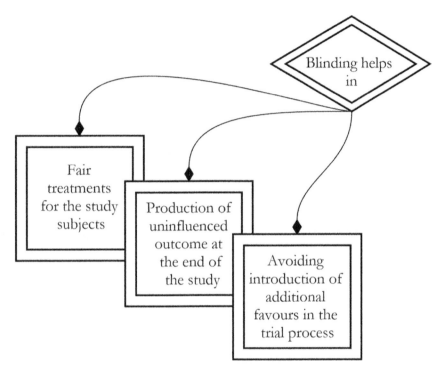

Fig: Advantages of blinding in clinical trial

To make blinding successful, enough care needs to be taken while deciding the intervention procedures so that the differences do not become the reason for unblinding. For example, in case of pharmacological trials, a placebo/standard treatment which is identical in appearance (for size, colour, weight, feel, odour etc.) and other aspects to the experimental treatment can be used to blind but this kind of blinding is hard to implement in case of non- pharmacological interventions (e.g., surgery).

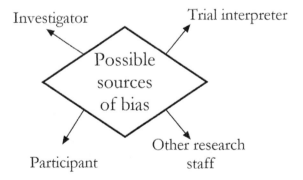

10.17 Types of blinding

Selection of the type of blinding depends on the need of the particular trial. **Fig – Types of blinding** explains the different types of blinding out of which investigator can select and can implement in his/her research.

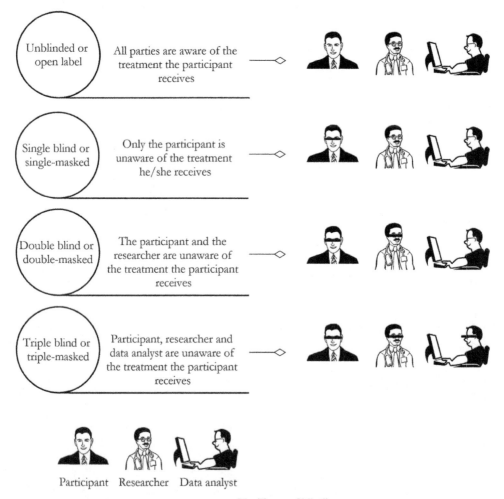

Fig: Types of blinding

However, the terms single-blind, double-blind and triple-blind do not have standard definitions. It means that there is no fixed rule about blinding of particular persons in a particular blinding type. For example - in a double-blind study, data analyst and subject can be unaware of the assigned treatments.

10.18 Unblinding (Code-break)

Blinding is used in a trial design to avoid the bias which can influence the research findings. But sometimes, blinding needs to be broken. This process is called "Unblinding".

Unblinding is the process by which the treatment/allocation details are made available either intentionally or unintentionally. Unblinding is the disclosure to the participant and/or study team regarding which treatment the participant is receiving during the trial.

Examples of unblinding

a)   When any unpleasant (toxic) event takes place in the trial, the site personnel may demand to break the code to know the actual treatment assignment so that the situation can be controlled.

b)   A study subject demands for disclosing of the actual treatment received during trial in order to act in his/her own best interest.

10.19 Types of Unblinding

Unblinding in a trial is a necessary process to protect participants in the event of any medical or safety issues. Unblinding can be of three types i.e., complete, partial and urgent unblinding (refer to the **Fig – Types of Unblinding**).

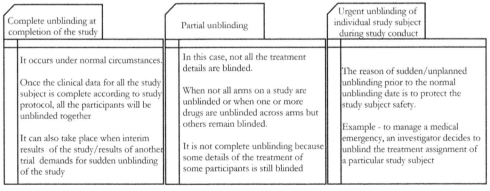

Fig: Types of Unblinding

10.20 Reasons for Unblinding

Typically, unblinding process occurs when the study team declares that all the data related to all the trial subjects is complete and clean.

Even though, unblinding which occurs before the fixed plan (according to the study protocol) may lead to error in the outcome of the study, it is sometimes imperative to do unblinding prior to the normal unblinding date (refer to the **Fig – Reasons for Unblinding**) due to some issues.

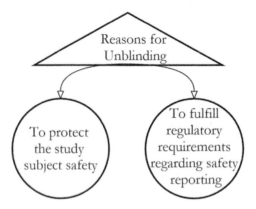

Fig: Reasons for Unblinding

All the details related to the process of unblinding are planned and documented in the study protocol, study specific standard operating procedures or in the study manual. There is also a defined process to 'break the blind' of a single participant when required. Research personnel should be well trained in the study specific unblinding procedures.

Chapter 11

SAFETY MONITORING OF A THERAPEUTIC PRODUCT

11.1 Learnings from the chapter

- *Safety concerns during drug development process*

- *The concept of pharmacovigilance with its process overview*

- *Few basic terms described (such as ADR, AE, SAE, expected and unexpected ADR)*

- *Types of reports and their reporting timeframes during clinical trial and post marketing space*

- *Basic overview of processing of adverse events/reactions during clinical trial and post marketing space*

- *Concept of SUSAR, Day zero and MSI*

11.2 Introduction

The therapeutic products manufactured with an intent to improve the public health may also produce adverse effects which must be monitored continuously during clinical trial (pre-approval/pre-marketing stage) and post clinical trial i.e., post marketing space (post approval/ marketing stage)

There should be continuous monitoring of safety aspects of a therapeutic product whether it is in the pre-market stage or post market stage. With continuous surveillance system, risks associated with the therapeutic products can be identified and controlled. However, the absence or any lack in the surveillance system of therapeutic product can lead to disasters.

The effects of healthcare products can be categorised as good effects and bad effects (refer to the **Fig- Effects of Healthcare products**).

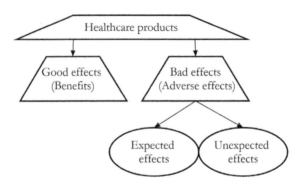

Fig: Effects of Healthcare products

Hence, it is important to improve the safety of the patient in terms of the use of medicines and this brings us to the topic of Pharmacovigilance.

11.3 Pharmacovigilance (PV)

Pharmacovigilance also known as Drug Safety, is defined as the science and activities relating to the detection, assessment, understanding and prevention of adverse effects or any other drug – related problem. Pharmacovigilance department ensures safe, rational and ethical use of drugs/ medicinal products.

11.4 Scope of Pharmacovigilance

Although the controlled clinical trials are considered as a hallmark of demonstrating the efficacy of a drug, safety data available from those trials have well recognized limitations, for example; limited number of study subjects included in the trial, limited duration of drug exposure, etc. These limitations make it imperative for the marketing authorization holder of a drug and the regulatory authority to continue with collecting, analysing and interpreting data relevant to patient safety that becomes available after the drug is introduced into the market.

Hence, Pharmacovigilance applies throughout the life cycle of a medicinal product. It applies to the pre-approval stage as much as it applies to the post-approval stage (refer to the **Fig – PV in pre & post authorization phases**).

11.5 Objectives of Pharmacovigilance

The contribution of medicine in human life is to improve the quality of life and the discipline of PV helps to achieve this. The important objectives of PV are depicted in **the Fig – Objectives of PV.**

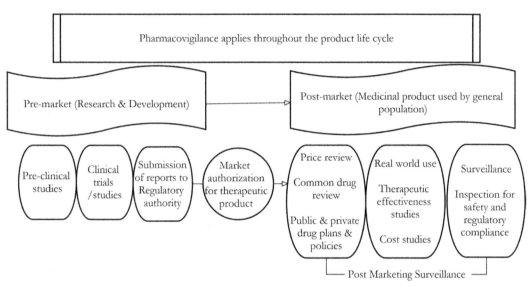

Fig: PV in pre & post authorization phases

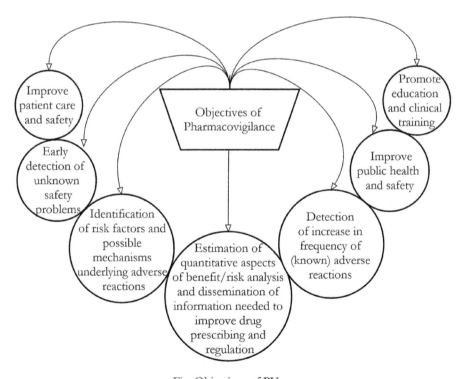

Fig: Objectives of PV

11.6 Tasks under Pharmacovigilance

Pharmacovigilance plays an important role in the life cycle of a medicinal product. It undertakes many roles for ensuring the safety of a medicinal product. Some of important roles are listed in the **Fig – Tasks under Pharmacovigilance.**

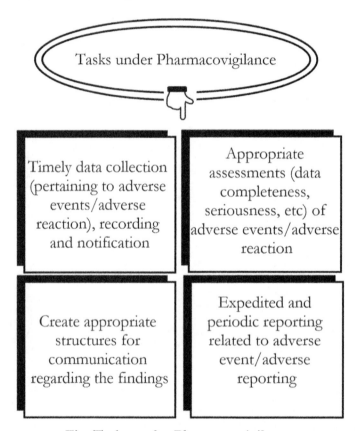

Fig: Tasks under Pharmacovigilance

Monitoring and reporting of adverse events correctly during a trial is one of the difficult tasks for investigator and other research staff. To follow a correct procedure for safety reporting, it is better to be clear about some basic concepts which are discussed below.

11.7 Adverse Drug Reaction (ADR)

Any substance that has a potential to produce therapeutic benefits, can be associated to some unwanted effects (mild to severe). For example, a person has taken a medicine for headache and he started feeling uneasiness and excessive sweating after having the medicine. Excessive sweating and uneasiness are the unwanted effects in this case.

Regarding pre-approval product in clinical experience:

All noxious and unintended responses to a medicinal product related to any dose should be considered adverse drug reactions (ADR).

The phrase "response to a medicinal product" means that a causal relationship between a medicinal product and an adverse event is at least a reasonable possibility, i.e., the relationship cannot be ruled out.

Regarding marketed medicinal products, according to WHO definition:

A response to a drug which is noxious and unintended and which occurs at doses normally used in human for prophylaxis, diagnosis or therapy of disease or for modification of physiological function.

11.8 Adverse Event (AE)

Adverse event is any untoward medical occurrence experienced by a patient (or a subject) who is administered with a medicinal product and does not necessarily having causal relationship with the treatment.

Hence, to quantify an AE, it is not necessary that a healthcare provider makes any determination about the causal link between the medical event and the drug exposure. An AE can therefore be any unfavourable and unintended sign (for example - abnormal laboratory findings), symptoms or disease which is temporally associated with the use of a medicinal product, whether considered related to the medicinal product or not considered related to the medicinal product.

11.9 ADR is a subset of AE

All Adverse Drug Reactions (ADRs) are Adverse Events (AEs) but all Adverse Events (AEs) are not Adverse Drug Reactions (ADRs).

The main difference between an adverse event (AE) and an adverse drug reaction (ADR) is that a causal relationship is suspected for the latter but is not required for the former. In this framework, adverse drug reactions are subset of adverse events. [Refer to **Fig – Adverse drug reaction (ADR) is the subset of adverse event (AE)**]

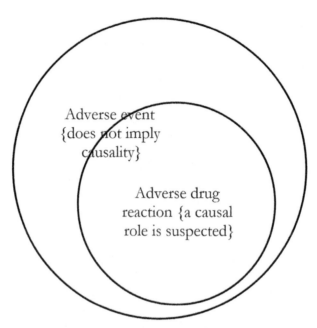

Fig: Adverse drug reaction (ADR) is
the subset of adverse event (AE)

11.10 Dimensions of Adverse Events

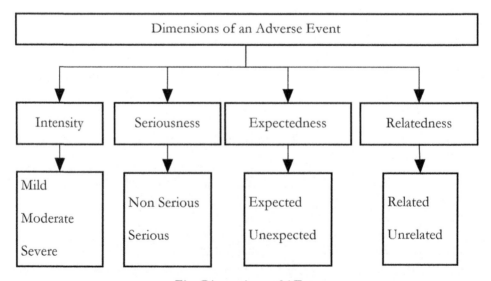

Fig: Dimensions of AE

The term "severe" is often used to describe the intensity (severity) of a specific event (as in mild, moderate or severe myocardial infarction). The event itself may be of relatively minor medical significance (such as severe headache) while the term "serious" is based on event outcome of the patient or the action criteria. Seriousness (not severity) serves as a guide for defining regulatory reporting obligations.

Serious	Severe
Defined as a regulatory definition	Defined as an intensity classification (mild, moderate, severe)

11.11 Serious Adverse Event (SAE)

Definition and Criteria of SAE

An adverse event is considered serious if it meets one or more of the following criteria

Death

Life threatening situation (Life threatening in the definition of a serious adverse event or serious adverse reaction refers to an event in which the patient/subject was at risk of death at the time of the event. It does not refer to an event which hypothetically might have caused death if it were more severe)

Requires inpatient hospitalization or prolongation of existing hospitalization

Disability (the condition of being unable to do things in the normal way)

Congenital anomalies/Birth defects (structural or functional anomalies including metabolic disorders which are present at the time of birth)

Important medical event (refers to which does not fit into other outcomes but require treatment to prevent one or the other outcomes. Example allergic bronchospasm (serious breathing problem) requires treatment in emergency room

11.12 Outcomes of SAE

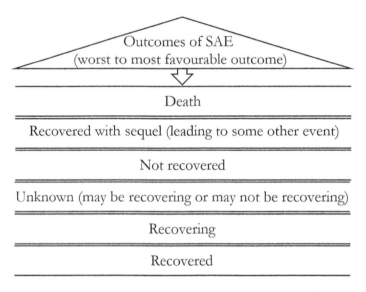

Outcomes of SAE
(worst to most favourable outcome)

Death
Recovered with sequel (leading to some other event)
Not recovered
Unknown (may be recovering or may not be recovering)
Recovering
Recovered

Note: Surgical procedures are not AEs/SAEs as per se, the condition for which surgical procedures are performed may be an AEs/SAEs which has to be reported. Surgical procedures are therapeutic measures of a condition requiring surgery. Surgical procedures planned prior to randomization and conditions leading to these measures are not AEs (this relates to medical history).

11.13 Expected ADR

Expected ADR refers to an ADR whose nature, severity, specificity, or outcome is consistent with the applicable product information (e.g., Investigator's Brochure for an unapproved investigational medicinal product/package insert or product monograph for marketed product).

11.14 Unexpected ADR

An unexpected ADR refers to the one whose nature, severity, specificity, or outcome is not consistent with the applicable product information (e.g., Investigator's Brochure for an unapproved investigational medicinal product/package insert or product monograph for marketed product).

When a Marketing Authorization Holder(MAH) is uncertain whether an ADR is expected or unexpected, the ADR should be treated as unexpected. An expected ADR with a fatal outcome should be considered unexpected unless the local/regional product labelling specifically states that the ADR might be associated with a fatal outcome.

11.15 Safety review throughout the drug development process

Throughout the clinical trials (pre-registration), safety is paramount. Review of safety is performed by R&D and pharmacovigilance departments within the sponsor companies. However, CROs (Contract Research Organization) is often contracted out clinical trial activities by the sponsor companies but the responsibility for safety lies with the sponsor company. In addition, safety may be reviewed continuously by independent Drug Safety Monitoring Boards set up for specific studies. The importance of safety in clinical research is depicted in the **Fig-Safety in drug development process**.

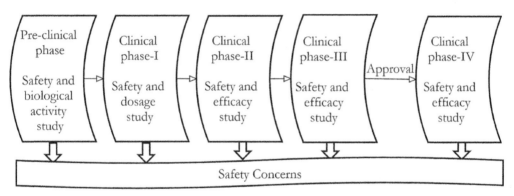

Fig: Safety in drug development process

11.16 Details of safety monitoring in a study protocol

The study protocol of any trial includes details regarding collection and handling of all the adverse events (serious and non-serious) which occur during a study. Some of the key elements related to safety monitoring which are included in the study protocol are mentioned in the **Fig – Details related to safety monitoring in a study protocol**.

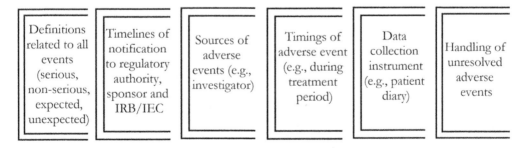

Fig: Details related to safety montoring in a study protocol

11.17 Basic flowchart of processing of adverse events/reactions during clinical trial

In the clinical trial process, when a subject experiences any adverse event/reaction, he/she informs to his/her investigator at clinical trial site, investigator reports this adverse event/reaction information to CRO and CRO reports the same to the PV department of pharmaceutical company (sponsor) for processing of adverse event/reaction and further company reports the adverse event/reaction information to the regulatory authority. In some cases, the investigator reports directly to Pharmaceutical company (in case no CRO in middle) [refer to the **Fig – Generalized process flow of adverse event/reaction during clinical trial**].

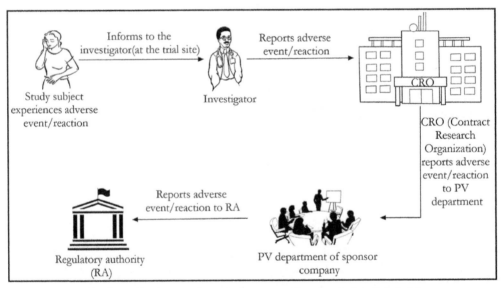

Fig: Generalized process flow of adverse event/reaction during clinical trial

11.18 Basic flowchart of processing of adverse events/reactions during post marketing space

In case of post marketing space, the patient informs adverse reaction to the health care professionals (HCP) such as physician/pharmacist/nurses/dentist/coroner (an official who holds inquest into violent, sudden and suspicious death), then the health care professional reports the ADR to the affiliates of pharmaceutical company and the affiliates inform the same to PV department of pharmaceutical company for further processing of ADR and reporting to the Regulatory authorities (refer to the **Fig – Generalized process flow of adverse event/reaction during post marketing space**).

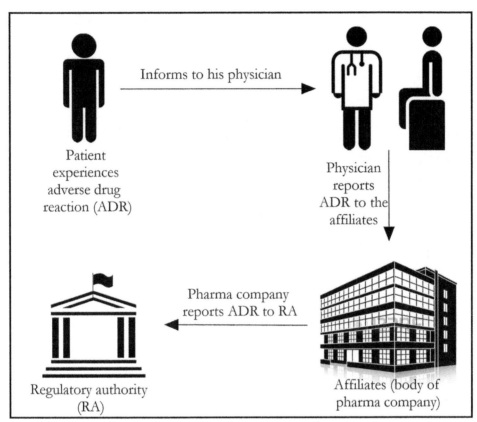

Fig: Generalized process flow of adverse event/reaction during post marketing space

11.19 What to Report (during clinical trial and post marketing space)

Reporting of adverse event/reaction during clinical trial and post marketing depends on various factors like seriousness, expectedness and causality. The following **Fig – What to Report** depicts the same.

Expedite means 'faster'. The ADRs which are unexpected, serious, fatal, & life threatening should be reported as fast as possible. Hence, these ADRs are subjected to expedited reporting. An expedited report would be a "Report" meeting the criteria for rapid transmission to a competent authority.

The purpose of expedited reporting is to make regulators, investigators, and other appropriate people aware of new, important information on serious reactions.

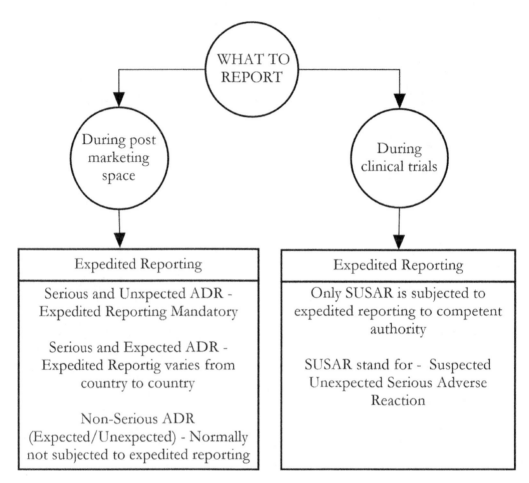

Fig: What to Report

During Clinical Trial

During clinical trial the causality assessment given by the investigator should not be downgraded by the sponsor. If the sponsor disagrees with the investigator's causality assessment, both the opinion of the investigator and that of the sponsor should be provided with the report. The expectedness of an adverse event/reaction shall be determined by the sponsor according to the reference document (refer to the **Fig – Assessment of Adverse event/reaction in terms of seriousness, causality and expectedness during clinical trial**). The reference document includes investigator's brochure for a non-authorized investigational medicinal product and summary of product characteristics (SmPC) for an authorized medicinal product.

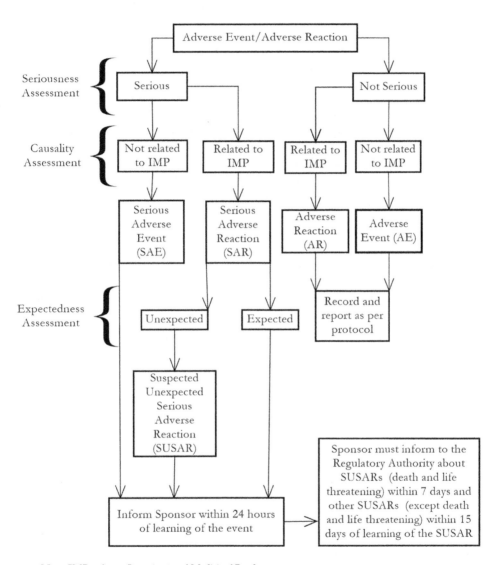

Note: IMP refers to Investigational Medicinal Product

Fig: Assessment of Adverse Event/Adverse Reaction in terms of seriousness, causality and expectedness during clinical trial

During clinical research with a medicinal product, there may be a causal link between the adverse reaction which occurs with subject and the medicinal product administered to the subject. This is known as SUSAR (SUSAR stands for Suspected Unexpected Serious Adverse Reaction) if the adverse reaction is both unexpected (not consistent with the applicable product information) and also meets the definition of a Serious Adverse Event/Reaction.

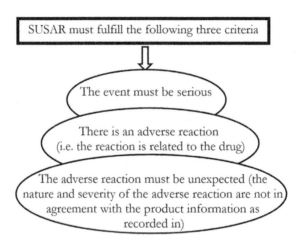

During Post marketing space

An ADR is the one which occurs at the normal doses when used for (a) diagnosis, (b) treatment, (c) precaution or (d) to explore the physiological functions and it is always related to drug. Hence, in case of PMS (Post marketing space) study, all the adverse effects should be reported as ADR.

11.20 Reporting Timeframe (during clinical trial and post marketing space)

Marketing Authorization Holder (MAH) is obliged to report about the adverse reaction/events to the regulatory authorities in a specific timeframe. In case the MAH is not compliant to this requirement, they would be facing some regulatory issues.

Reporting of SUSAR during Clinical trial

In a clinical trial, SUSARs which are life-threatening or have fatal consequences, must be reported to the regulatory authority and to the IRB/IEC at the latest (within 7 calendar days of the sponsor becoming aware of them). All relevant information on the aftermath of this SUSAR must be reported within a time frame of a further 8 days. Other reports of SUSARs must be prepared within 15 calendar days (India- 14 calendar days) of the sponsor becoming aware of them.

The investigator at the clinical trial site however, should inform all SAE (except those adverse events, which the protocol and other relevant documents identify as not needing immediate reporting) immediately (within 24 hrs of knowing about the SAE) to the sponsor and to the Ethics Committee within 7 working days (refer to the **Fig – Reporting timeframe during clinical trial**).

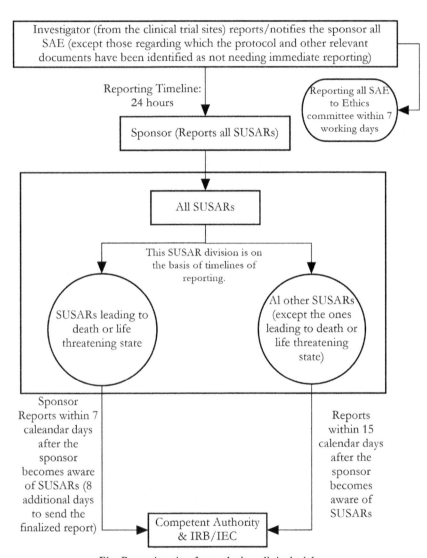

Fig: Reporting timeframe during clinical trial

Reporting timeframe during post marketing space

Reporter (e.g., patient's relative, physician) can report the ADRs related to a medicinal product directly to the company which is marketing the product, or to the regulatory authority. However, the MAH has to report all serious ADR (under legal obligation) to health authority within 15 calendar days of becoming aware of ADR (refer to the **Fig –Reporting timeframe during post marketing space**).

The Regulatory reporting time clock is considered to start on the date when any personnel of MAH (Marketing Authorization Holder) first receives a case report that fulfils the minimum criteria as well as the criteria of expedited reporting. This date should be considered as "Day 0".

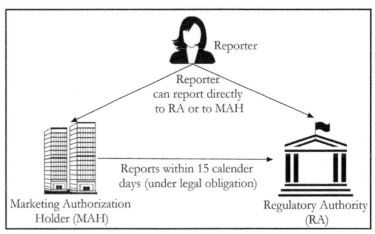

Fig: Reporting timeframe during post marketing space

11.21 Day Zero

Day zero is the date on which any personnel of an organization (MAH) or the third party which has a contractual agreement with that organization, receives the case report/adverse reaction report (for the first time) that fulfills the minimum criteria as well as the criteria of expedited reporting.

Example: A patient reports an adverse reaction with only 3 MSI (Minimum Safety Information) out of 4 MSI elements to a manufacturer on 5th June 2017 and gives 4th element of MSI on 9th June 2017. In this case, 9th June will be considered as Day Zero as report meets the criteria of valid report with 4 elements of MSI on 9th June.

If a CRO which is in contract with a pharma company (manufacturer) for managing its drug safety activities and this CRO receives information about an adverse reaction from a health care professional on 10th May 2017, then in this case Day Zero will be considered 10th May 2017 as CRO is in a contract with the manufacturer.

11.22 MSI – Minimum Safety Information

According to WHO criteria, there is a set of basic information required before a case report becomes acceptable. The criteria are mentioned in the **Fig – MSI**.

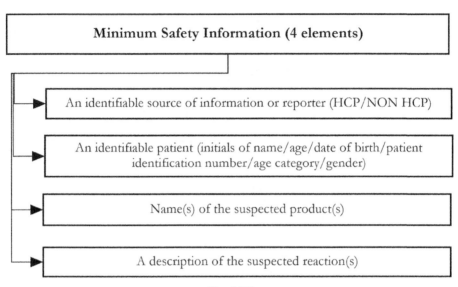

Minimum Safety Information (4 elements)

An identifiable source of information or reporter (HCP/NON HCP)

An identifiable patient (initials of name/age/date of birth/patient identification number/age category/gender)

Name(s) of the suspected product(s)

A description of the suspected reaction(s)

Fig: MSI

The four elements (mentioned in the Fig: MSI) are called Minimum Safety Information (MSI) which makes any report valid for pharmacovigilance database. MSI helps in avoiding duplication of cases, detection of fraudulence and also helps in facilitating the follow up process.

If one or more of these four elements are missing, the case is not considered a valid AE report. Although there are no exceptions to this rule, but there may be situation that may require a judgment call. For example, the term "identifiable" may not always be clear-cut. If a physician reports that he/she has a patient "A" taking drug "X" who experienced an AE, but the physician refuses to provide any specifics about patient "A", then the report is still a valid case even though the patient is not specifically identified. This is because the reporter has first-hand information about the patient and the patient is identifiable (i.e. a real person) to the physician.

Note: In different countries and regions of the world, drugs are sold under various trade names.

11.23 Pharmacovigilance process overview

Case processing is a processing of ADR reports that the company receives from various sources. The steps of case processing have been summarized below:

• Once the case of adverse event/reaction is received from any source (telephone, fax, email, forms, regulators, etc), the case is checked for 4 valid criteria i.e., minimum safety information (MSI).

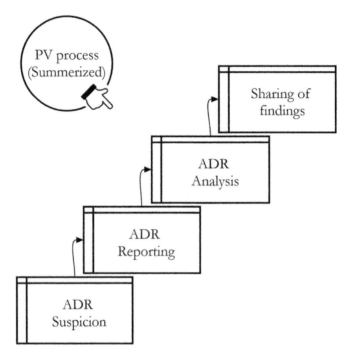

- If the case is valid, the adverse event/reaction coding is done using standardized terminology from MedDRA and then the case is evaluated for its seriousness criteria by triage team.

- A unique identity number is assigned to each individual case.

- Then, the case is sent to the safety associate for data entry. The work of case processing team starts now.

- The safety associate enters the case details into safety database, performs coding (for disease and medicine) and writes narratives of the case.

- In case of any query, he/she seeks the follow up information from the reporter.

- After the data entry, the case is assigned to the QC (quality control) team where the QC person checks the work done by safety associates.

- The case moves in the workflow to the Medical Reviewer who assesses the medical aspects of the case, performs the causality assessment (relationship of given ADR and specific drug) and gives a company comment on each case.

- Next step is Signal detection (identifying signals i.e. potential indicator of new ADR) and Risk Management Plan (risk assessment and risk minimization plan) post which the analysis is completed through various methods like statistical methods (e.g. t-test for the comparison of mean), data manipulation (e.g. tabular and graphics).

- Now the case is ready for submission to the regulatory authority and for communication to other partners. The submission team submits the case to regulatory agencies according to the local requirements.

The case processing steps are depicted in the **Fig – PV overview (generalized).**

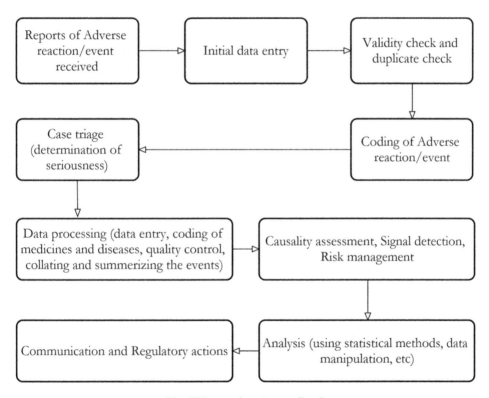

Fig: PV overview (generalized)

Causality assessment: - evaluation of the likelihood that a particular treatment is the cause of an observed adverse event

Signal detection: - process of identification of relation between drug and adverse event/reaction.

{For detail knowledge on Pharmacovigilance please refer the book "Mind maps of pharmacovigilance basics"}

Chapter 12

CLINICAL DATA MANAGEMENT

12.1 Learnings from the chapter

- *Introduction to Clinical Data Management (CDM) including its importance and objectives*

- *Role of CDM during a clinical trial process*

- *Details of different aspects such as data entry, discrepancy management, query management, SAE reconciliation, database lock, report creation, data transfer, etc.*

- *Notes on DMP (data management plan)*

- *Key players of CDM department*

12.2 Introduction

A huge amount of data is collected during the whole process of a clinical trial. All the data generated as a result of the trial related activities is called "clinical data". Integrity and quality of clinical data is very crucial for drug developers as the approval process of an investigational product by the regulatory authorities totally depends on this data. Hence, management of clinical data is an essential part of clinical research.

12.3 Clinical Data Management (CDM)

Clinical data management is a multi-disciplinary activity. It includes collection of all clinical data during the trial process and then the collected data is reviewed and analysed to produce quality data that can be considered reliable (refer to the **Fig – Data management process**). In simple words, Clinical data management is the collection, integration and validation of clinical data.

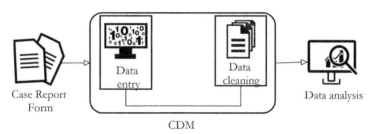

Fig: Data management process

Clinical data management is a critical aspect in clinical research as it generates high-quality, reliable, and statistically sound data from clinical trials by keeping the number of errors and missing data as low as possible and by gathering maximum data for the analysis. High-quality data refers to the data which comply with protocol specifications and are accurate and suitable for statistical analysis.

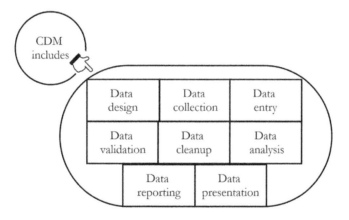

12.4 Objectives of Clinical Data Management

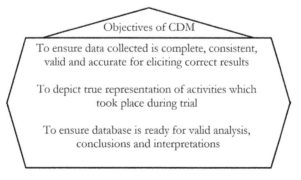

12.5 Importance of Clinical Data Management

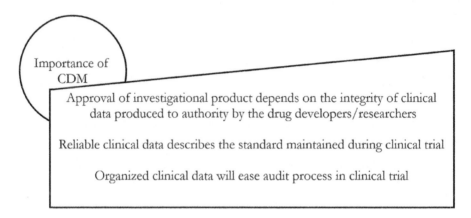

12.6 Collection of Clinical data

Clinical data (during clinical trial process) can be gathered from various sources (refer to the **Fig – Collection of clinical data**).

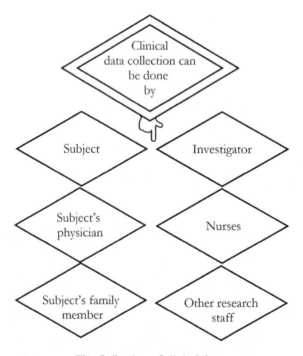

Fig: Collection of clinical data

12.7 Key members and their respective roles in CDM

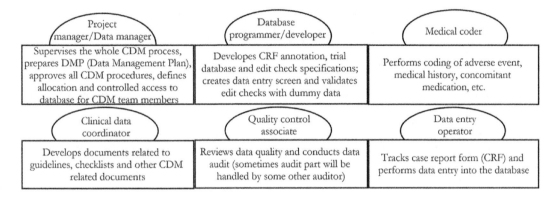

Project manager/Data manager	Database programmer/developer	Medical coder
Supervises the whole CDM process, prepares DMP (Data Management Plan), approves all CDM procedures, defines allocation and controlled access to database for CDM team members	Developes CRF annotation, trial database and edit check specifications; creates data entry screen and validates edit checks with dummy data	Performs coding of adverse event, medical history, concomitant medication, etc.
Clinical data coordinator	Quality control associate	Data entry operator
Develops documents related to guidelines, checklists and other CDM related documents	Reviews data quality and conducts data audit (sometimes audit part will be handled by some other auditor)	Tracks case report form (CRF) and performs data entry into the database

12.8 Data flow in clinical trial

Clinical data during a clinical trial touches many hands and crosses many steps to reach the destination. The flow of clinical data in a trial has been depicted in the **Fig- Data flow in a clinical trial**.

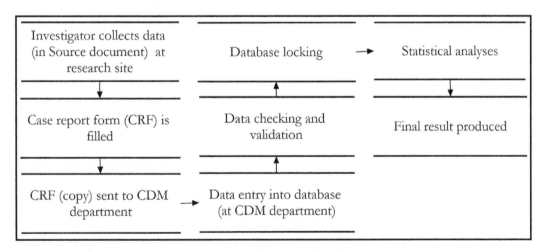

Fig: Data flow in a clinical trial

12.9 Data Management Plan (DMP)

DMP describes the database structure and the procedures that should be used for system testing and validation. It also explains procedures for data entry, edit checks, data coding, data queries and query resolution. This document is based on study protocol, CRF and CRF instructions. DMP is needed to be updated when there is any protocol amendment or change in data handling process.

12.10 Objectives of DMP

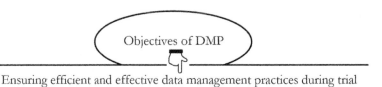

Ensuring efficient and effective data management practices during trial

Detailing about all data management activities and respective roles and responsibilities of personnel involved in data management activities

Ensuring correctness and accuracy of data collected during trial for eliciting valid results and conclusions from the study

12.11 Benefits of DMP

Benefits of DMP	Ensures compliance with good clinical data management practices throughout the trial
	Serves as a document which will be helpful in proper planning, training, communication and execution of data management activities
	Personnel involved in data management activities become aware of their respective roles and responsibilities which enhance the smoothness of process
	Provides continuity for data management activities when personnel in data management team changes
	Provides a record of data handling activities by different individuals during study
	Assures production of quality data during trial

12.12 DMP components

DMP details about project specifications (such as data specification, data processing, timelines, data edit checks, etc.) which are needed to be implemented during a clinical trial (refer to the **Fig – DMP components**).

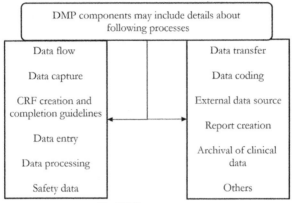

Fig: DMP components

12.13 Role of CDM in clinical trial

Clinical data management department participates in every bit of the trial as this department is responsible for producing quality clinical data. Important roles of CDM in a clinical trial is described in the **Fig – Role of CDM in clinical trial.**

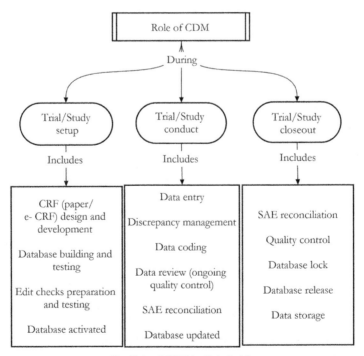

Fig: Role of CDM in clinical trial

12.14 Trial/study setup

During study setup, CDM department gets involved in the designing and development of CRF, database building and testing and edit checks preparation and their testing. All of these have been explained below.

Trial/study Setup

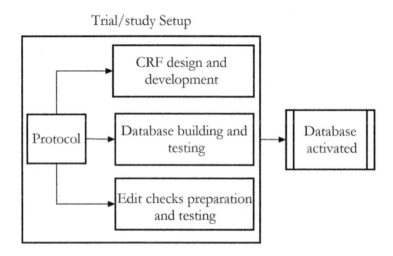

12.15 CRF design and development

Clinical data quality relies on the quality of data collection instrument i.e. Case Report Form (CRF). CRF is a document where the investigator enters all the data (clinical and non- clinical) of a study subject (who is related to a particular trial). It contains data related to patient's health parameters and the data related to medical procedures performed during trial.

CRF should be concise, user friendly and self-explanatory. Sponsor's input is required for correction and approval of final version of CRF. Before designing the CRF, final protocol should be handy as CRF translates protocol-specific activities into data being generated. Data field should be clearly defined in CRF and the type of data to be entered should be evident from the CRF. For example, if weight has to be captured in two decimal places, the data entry field should have two data boxes placed after the decimal as shown in fig below:

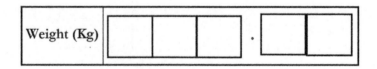

CRF annotation is the first step in translating CRF into a database application. Annotations are "coded terms" which are used in CDM to indicate the variables in the study. CDM annotates the CRFs by establishing variable names for each item to be entered. Annotated CRF tells where the data collected for each question is stored in the database. (An annotated CRF is a blank CRF with markings/annotations that coordinate each point in the form with its corresponding dataset name).

12.16 Types of CRF (Paper CRF and e- CRF)

CRF can be Paper CRF or e-CRF (electronic CRF). Few important features related to these two types of CRFs are mentioned below:

Features of Paper CRF and e-CRF

Features	Paper CRF	Electronic CRF (e - CRF)
Time required for data entry	More	Less
Number of discrepancies	More	Less (due to in built edit checks)
Query resolution	Slow	Fast
Time taken to complete and analyze	More	Less
Chances of error	Higher	Lower
Accuracy	Less	More
Data management	Tedious	Improved

12.17 Database building and testing

Database is a structured set of data (rows, column). Clinical data is collected and stored in Clinical Data Management System (CDMS). Example – Excel spreadsheet, RAVE, Clintrial, Oracle Clinical, InForm, etc.

12.18 Features of CDMS (Clinical Data Management System)

Quality and integrity of clinical database plays an important role in the success of clinical trial. Some desirable features of CDMS are listed in **Fig – Desirable features of CDMS**.

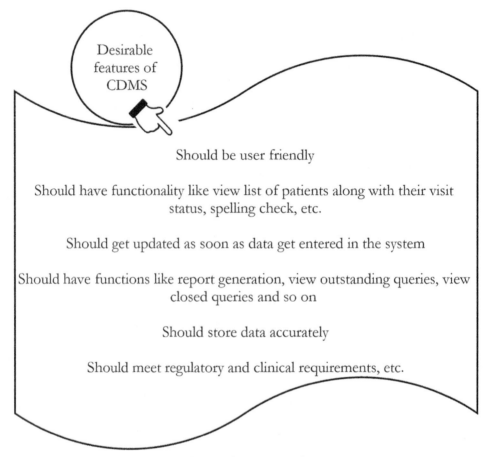

Fig: Desirable features of CDMS

According to regulations, the functioning of CDMS must be tested before introducing the newly built database to the live study. It will be tested by entering dummy data in the test sites (non-study data environment) in order to check if it is functioning as intended. Any changes in structure/programming must be tested and performed first in test site before using it in the "production (a study site environment)" database. Once the database is reviewed and fully tested, it will be used in live study where the study data will be entered.

12.19 Edit checks preparation and testing

Edit check is a program instruction that tests the validity of input in a data entry program. For example, if the entry on Gender field is 'Male', there should not be data for pregnancy test result field.

12.20 Edit checks

Edit specifications list is a document which contains details of all edit checks (refer to the **Fig – Kinds of edit checks**) i.e. which data shall be checked and queried (if necessary). The edit checks are programmed according to this edit check list and the programming starts with the sponsor's approval to this list. Test subjects are entered in the database to test the entry screens and to test the programming. It is important that every check produces either positive or negative proof at least once.

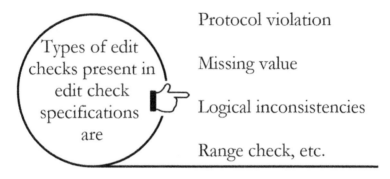

Fig: Kinds of edit checks

Effective implementation of edit check can prevent the illogical, incomplete, or inconsistent data from being entered into the database, which will further make the data analyses much easier.

12.21 Trial/study conduct

The various roles of CDM team during conduct of the trial has been described below in detail.

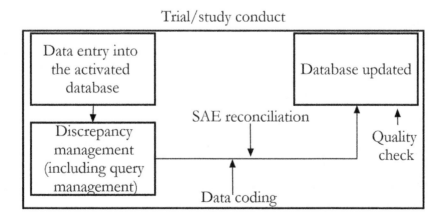

The activated database is ready to receive the data. To do data entry from the case report form (CRF) to the CDM system, it is important to track all CRF in the study process.

12.22 CRF tracking

CRF (paper/electronic) tracking is the process of knowing the state in which the page is existing currently in the data management process. CRF workflow describes the path followed by the pages and the states the pages are in. Few common states of CRF workflow are listed in the **Fig – States of CRF workflow**.

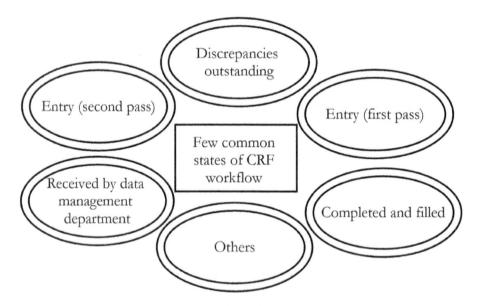

Fig: States of CRF workflow

Clinical Research Associate (CRA) monitors the entries which are made in the CRF to ensure completeness of the CRF. Completed CRFs will be retrieved and handed over to the CDM team. The CDM team will track the retrieved CRFs and will maintain their record. CRFs are tracked for missing pages and illegible data manually to assure that the data is not lost. In case of missing or illegible data, a clarification is obtained from the investigator and the issue is resolved. Tracking of CRF may take time in handling some typical unwanted situations (refer to the **Fig – Undesirable situations encountered during tracking of CRF**).

The main objective of CRF tracking is to ensure that all the data is present in complete form and no information is missing. Proper tacking of CRF leads to less time consumption in administrative process and aids in generating quality data.

Duplicate page (e.g., investigative site staff filled out a CRF incorrectly but already data collected in that form and again a new form is filled with same content but with corrections)

Pages with no data (e.g., patient missed visit and so the pages in CRF designed for that visit will be blank)

Repeating pages with the same page number (i.e., more than one copy of a page with same page number)

Pages without page number, etc.

Fig: Undesirable situations encountered during tracking of CRF

12.23 Data entry

It is a process of entering /transferring data from CRF to clinical data management system (CDMS). There are several methods (refer to the **Fig – Methods of data entry**) available for data entry. The drug developer can choose the method of data entry in accordance with their set objectives. Data entry can be done manually or it can be done by use of OCR (Optical Character Recognition) system.

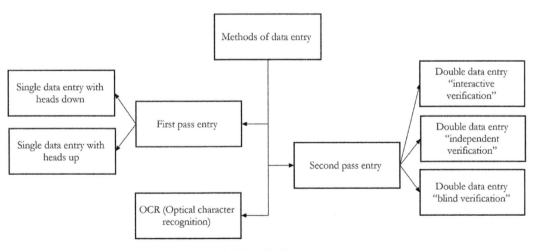

Fig: Methods of data entry

The various methods of data entry have been explained below:

12.24 First pass entry

This refers to the data being entered in the database for the first time. Different types of first pass entry are depicted in the **Fig – Types of First pass entry**.

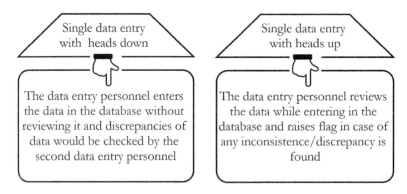

Fig: Types of First pass entry

12.25 Second pass entry

This refers to data being entered by second data entry personnel following the first data entry. An alert gets notified by the system in case second personnel enters something different from first entry. Different types of second pass entry are depicted in the **Fig – Types of Second pass entry**.

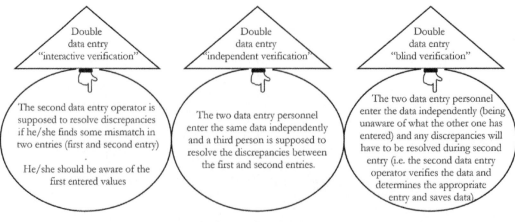

Fig Types of Second pass entry

12.26 OCR (Optical Character Recognition)

It is a method in which software converts scanned image to machine readable and editable text. The software recognizes the characters from paper CRF or e-CRF and these data would be placed directly into the database. Data entered through OCR method need to be checked for accuracy.

12.27 Data capture

Whether a trial is small or large, it is important for the organization to collect and manage the clinical data accurately, efficiently and in compliance with regulations. Data capture can be defined as a collection of clinically significant data during the trials in order to process the data for generating reports for the regulatory submission for various purposes. It can be of two types (Refer to **Fig – Types of data capture**).

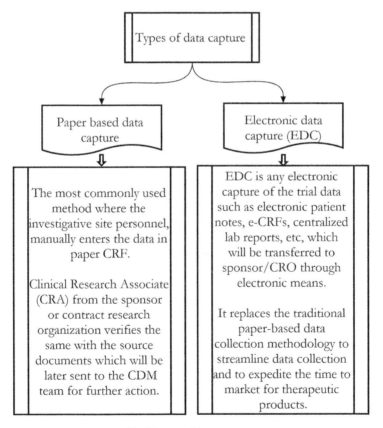

Fig: Types of data capture

12.28 Discrepancy management

It is a cleaning process of discrepancies present in clinical data of CDMS using edit checks (manual checks/electronic checks). It is also known as" data cleaning" or "data validation" process which is used to assure validity and accuracy of data.

12.29 Data cleaning

Data cleaning can be done manually or through electronic means (refer to the **Fig – Data cleaning methods**).

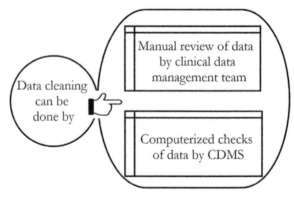

Fig: Data cleaning methods

12.30 Benefits of data cleaning

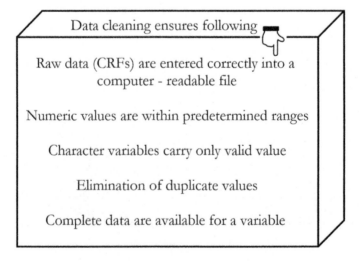

12.31 Checklist for data cleaning

Data cleaning can be performed with the help of a checklist (list of checks that need to be performed) [refer to the **Fig – Checklist for data cleaning**]. This helps to create quality data and to eliminate the chances of missing any important activities.

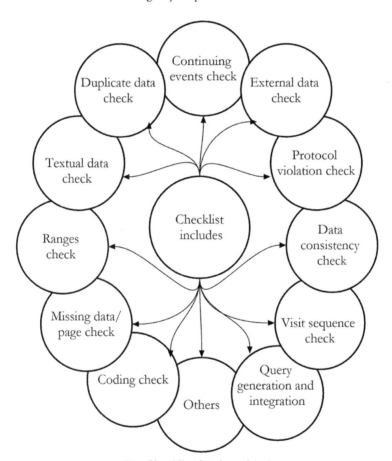

Fig: Checklist for data cleaning

12.32 Process of resolving discrepancies

Discrepancies are any inconsistencies in the clinical data which need to be resolved.

Discrepancies are generated once the validation procedures (edit checks) are applied to the entered data. CDM system which store discrepancies, tracks its status, records its resolution and lists the type of resolution is known as "Discrepancy management system".

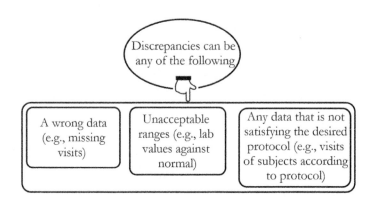

Discrepancies can be resolved by the data management team at sponsor/CRO place. But if there is any doubt, the query will be sent to the investigative site through data clarification form (DCF) via paper/electronic mode. In case of electronic process, the query can be generated automatically with the help of edit checks, which identifies the value which is not according to specified protocol. For better query management, it is advisable to identify the origin of discrepancies (refer to the **Fig – Process of resolving discrepancies**).

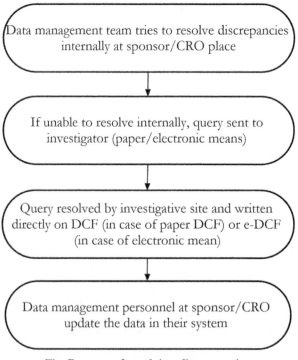

Fig: Process of resolving discrepancies

12.33 Query management process

The query management steps are listed below:

- Query is created by the data management team and it is sent to the investigator

- In case of no response, same response, inconsistence response, incorrect or incomplete response, re-query is required

- Data management team keeps a track and proper documentation of the flow of query between investigative site and data management team

- Types of query resolution - The various types of query resolution are mentioned in the **Fig – Types of query resolution**.

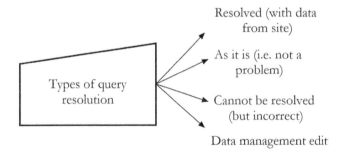

Fig: Types of query resolution

- Arrangement of query text - first mention the location of query, then state the discrepancy (issue) and then ask for resolution (Refer to **Fig – Formula for query writing**).

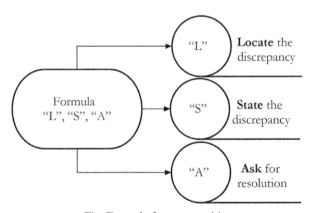

Fig: Formula for query writing

• Query Status – It states the state of query raised by the data management team. The different types of query status have been depicted in the **Fig – Types of query status**.

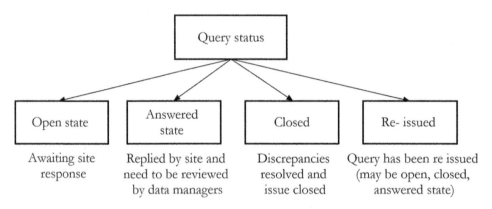

Fig: Types of query status

12.34 Data (Medical) coding

Clinical data can be generated at various clinical trial sites by different research teams in various countries. Hence, medical coding is required to maintain uniformity in medical terms to ease the whole process of trial. Coding of clinical data into a standardized terminology facilitates its analysis. Medical coders categorize the medical terms reported appropriately so that they can be analysed and reviewed easily.

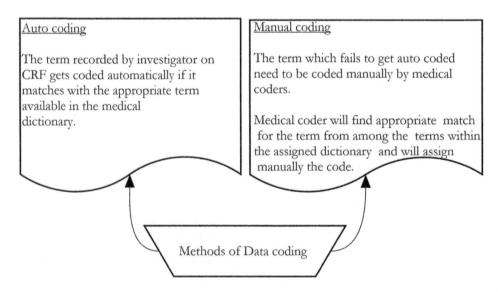

Some terms may not be clear to the medical coder for coding purpose. In that case, a query will be sent to investigator/ medically qualified expert for clarification. Based on the resolution received from the investigator/ medically qualified experts, medical coder will do the coding with appropriate code.

Medical coding for a study is done as per the project specific protocol requirement. Most commonly used dictionaries are MedDRA i.e. Medical Dictionary for Regulatory Activities and WHODD i.e. World Health Organization Drug Dictionary.

12.35 SAE Reconciliation

An adverse event, which occurs during the conduct of a clinical trial, is needed to be collected in clinical database as well as in safety database (refer to the **Fig – Handling process of SAE data**). The purpose of collection of events in safety database is to ensure that the serious adverse events are reported quickly. It is important for the clinical data manager to ensure that data is reconciled between these two databases.

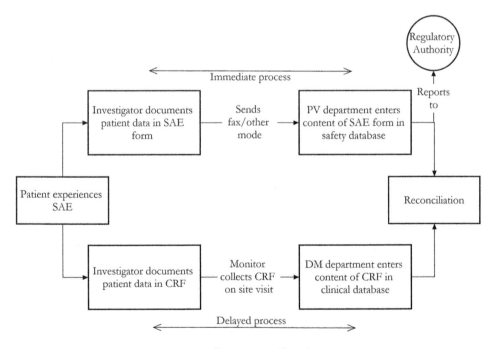

Fig: Handling process of SAE data

SAE (Serious Adverse Event) reconciliation process allows the comparison of key safety data variables between CDMS and pharmacovigilance (PV) system to ensure that the data is consistent and not contradictory in two databases (refer to the **Fig – Data required for reconciliation process**).

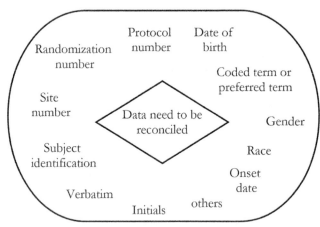

Fig: Data required for reconciliation process

While comparing the key safety data, it is important to check the following:

* Key safety data fields are same (in both electronic and manual comparison)
* Key safety data is in the same format
* Key safety data share the same value code list for the same field

12.36 When to perform SAE reconciliation

It is a frequentative process which occurs several times during the trial. The occurrence of this process may depend on the multiple factors. Some of the important factors are mentioned in the **Fig – Factors deciding occurrence of SAE reconciliation**.

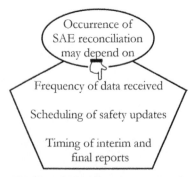

Fig: Factors deciding occurrence of
SAE reconciliation

12.37 SAE reconciliation process overview

SAE reconciliation process needs the SAE reconciliation plan. This process is performed by the data management team with the support of pharmacovigilance department (refer to the **Fig – Pharmacovigilance department & Clinical data management department**).

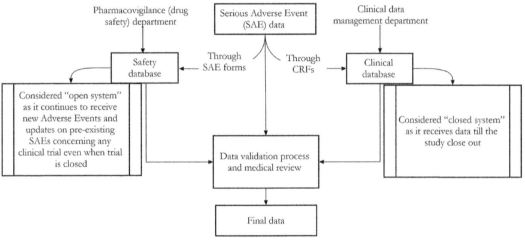

Fig: Pharmacovigilance department & Clinical data management department

Cut – off point - The SAEs reporting continues even after the trial ends. Hence, it is important to fix a cut-off point, post which no SAEs or updates will be added to the clinical database so that the processes will be considered closed for clinical database, however, the safety database will continue to receive SAEs and updates concerning that particular clinical trial.

Pre –requisite of SAE Reconciliation

Prior to the reconciliation process, it is the responsibility of clinical data management team to ensure that all the Pre –requisites of SAE Reconciliation are fulfilled (refer to the **Fig – Pre – requisite of SAE reconciliation**).

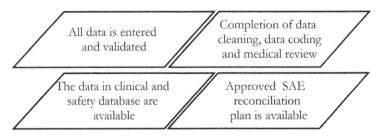

Fig: Pre requisite of SAE Reconciliation

Basically, the clinical and safety database are compared for consistency and exact matches using manual or electronic processes. The main objective of this process is to compare the SAE in clinical database with SAE in safety database to ensure the quality of SAE data in a trial. Data manager combines the two SAE tables from two databases into SAE reconciliation and sends to the scientist for review.

Steps involved in SAE reconciliation

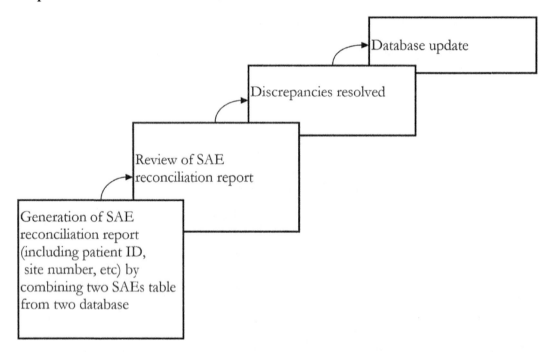

Fig: SAE reconciliation process-summarized

The steps involved in SAE reconciliation have been explained below:

- Generation of SAE reconciliation report – The data from two (clinical and safety) database is extracted to create the two lists for direct comparison.

- Review of SAE reconciliation report - Cross checking of the number of events in each database is done. This process checks if the number of events are same in both the databases. This process also verifies that each entry of SAE in safety database is flagged as an SAE in clinical database and vice versa (Note: some SAEs in safety database may not be present in clinical database until all CRFs are collected and entered). SAEs which are present in the clinical database but not in the safety database must be documented as these are potentially unreported events but they should go to safety team. Similarly, SAEs present in the safety database but absent in the clinical database should be reviewed. According to the plan, key data should be compared in each database.

- Discrepancies resolved - All the differences between SAEs present in both the databases should be reviewed and resolved. Query inconsistencies also need a review according to the plan. Depending upon the nature of discrepancy, intervention by medical monitor may be required before reaching to any decision.

- Database update – Database will be updated with signed and dated responses.

12.38 Purpose of SAE Reconciliation

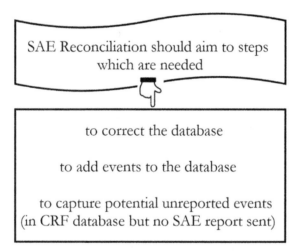

SAE Reconciliation should aim to steps which are needed

to correct the database

to add events to the database

to capture potential unreported events (in CRF database but no SAE report sent)

12.39 Quality control

Accurate clinical data can be a proof of a safe and effective drug. Hence, it is imperative to assure the quality of clinical data as it is going to decide the fate of an investigational product. The basic features which should be present in a quality data are mentioned in the **Fig – Basic elements of quality data.**

Quality can be maintained throughout the study by performing quality checks at certain intervals for all critical and non-critical data points before locking the database. This step ensures that the produced data is accurate, credible, clean and correct. In the absence of proper quality check process, there are chances of getting some error which may be unseen/unobserved/undetected and which ultimately leads to a systematic error in data analyses and in the eliciting conclusions at the end of the study.

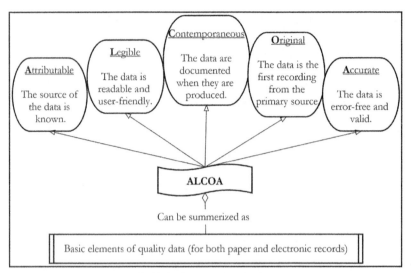

Fig: Basic elements of quality data

Double data entry is considered as the first quality check to ensure that data entry is done correctly and CRFs are transcribed accurately in the system. CRFs are considered as raw data and the quality and accuracy of database can be checked against CRFs and the associated Data Clarification Forms (DCFs). In case of electronic version, the transcribed data will be checked against e-CRFs.

12.40 Database Security and Data Storage

Clinical data produced from clinical trial are supposed to have limited access and should be stored in a secured environment as the integrity and the quality of data is a very important concern for the regulatory agency. Actions taken towards security of database are listed in the **Fig – Database security**.

The access to CDMS will be of different degrees for different personnel. For example – data entry person will get access only for data entry of the data related to his/her particular project; the discrepancy manager can only raise query and cannot make any changes/modification to the data.

Data storage is an important step in clinical trial as these data may be required for future references. Data should be stored in the same platform in which it was locked for easy availability. Suppose data was locked in Oracle platform then it should be archived on a compatible version of Oracle for easy access. The archived data will be separate from production data and hence the handling of archived data will be done separately.

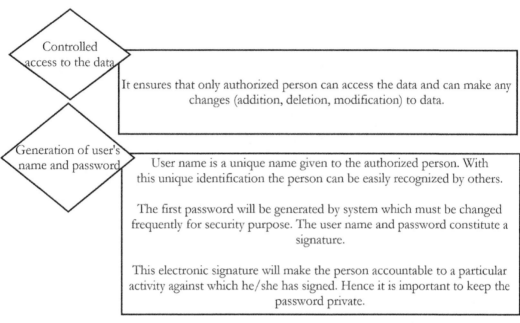

Controlled access to the data

It ensures that only authorized person can access the data and can make any changes (addition, deletion, modification) to data.

Generation of user's name and password

User name is a unique name given to the authorized person. With this unique identification the person can be easily recognized by others.

The first password will be generated by system which must be changed frequently for security purpose. The user name and password constitute a signature.

This electronic signature will make the person accountable to a particular activity against which he/she has signed. Hence it is important to keep the password private.

Fig: Database security

Data storage may include audit trail (tells who did what), database design, coding details, derived values, etc.

12.41 Trial/Study closeout

Trial/Study closeout

SAE reconciliation (Final)		Database release
Quality control	Database Lock	Data storage

12.42 Database lock

Once the last patient's final visit is done at the trial site, it is desired by sponsor to lock the database as soon as possible so that the analysis process can start for eliciting the conclusions of the study. Once the data is locked, no manipulation can be done in it during analysis.

Sometimes, after locking data, there may be a requirement for some changes in the data (for example- the missing data need to be filled). For making changes in data, the database has to be unlocked and post making the changes, the database must be relocked. Unlocking of database depends on factors such as (a) how important or critical it is to make the changes in the locked data or (b) there are many changes required in locked data which can impact the analysis.

12.43 Review of data quality

Sponsor prefers to finish all the required activities before locking the database in order to attain the high quality of clinical data because unlocking and relocking are not simple steps. There are different kinds of close review which can be helpful in assuring the quality of data (refer to the **Fig – Review steps to assure data quality**).

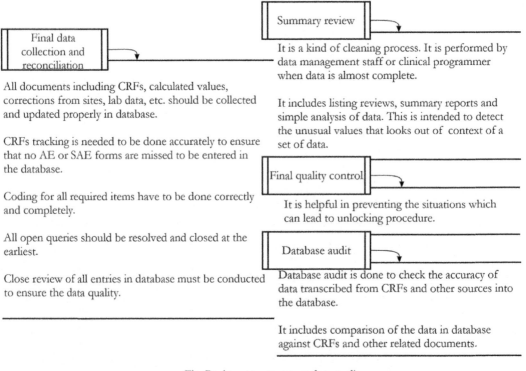

Fig: Review steps to assure data quality

Locking of Database

Once all the pre-activities to database lock are completed, the database will be set to get locked. Database lock means data is clean and ready for analysis and any amendment, deletion or update to database is not possible hereafter. There are two types of database lock (refer to the **Fig** – **Types of database lock**).

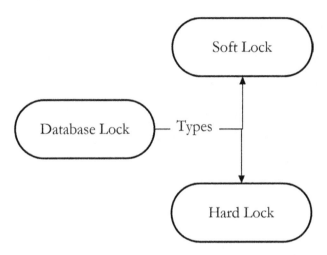

Fig: Types of database lock

12.44 Soft lock

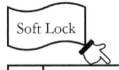

	The soft lock is the intimation to start database audit and final quality check for quality assurance. Edit rights are taken away from clinical data management team and only the project manager or the database administrator of the project may have right to edit/modify which would be captured in audit trail. Some companies call the point at which the last CRF comes in from the research site as "Soft lock" or "Freeze" while some other companies prefer to wait until the last query resolution to receive to declare the soft lock.

12.45 Hard lock

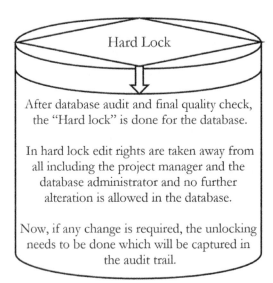

Hard Lock

After database audit and final quality check, the "Hard lock" is done for the database.

In hard lock edit rights are taken away from all including the project manager and the database administrator and no further alteration is allowed in the database.

Now, if any change is required, the unlocking needs to be done which will be captured in the audit trail.

12.46 Unlocking of Database

Once the database is locked, the analysis process starts. During the analysis process, if the programmer finds some problem with the data (which needs corrections), he/she calls for unlocking. Unlocking of database for resolving the problem need a detailed review of reasons by the upper management prior to unlocking the database. Database will be unlocked only if the assessor feels that the changes required are substantial. Appropriate quality control, review and approval will be required again to relock the database.

12.47 Re-locking of database

Once the required changes are done, relocking of database will have to be performed following the same standard operating procedure of locking.

Once the database is locked, it will be released to statistical team for analysis to draw out conclusions. Study files and documents should be properly archived and backed up.

12.48 Report creation and data transfer

Types of report

There can be requirements of different types of reports for different reasons such as for data management review, data evaluation, decision making regarding safety and efficacy of an intervention, administrative purposes, etc. Most often, the data management (DM) team is asked to create these reports which can be used by the different players of the trial. These reports can be of two types (refer to the **Fig – Types of reports created by data management team**).

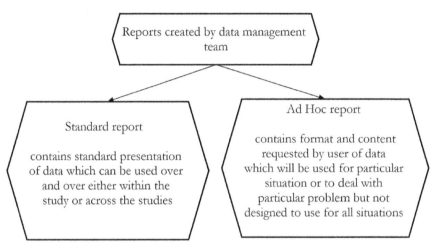

Fig:Types of reports created by data management team

Data transfer

Data transfer (internally/externally) also comes under the umbrella of the DM team. For instance, the DM personnel is asked to transfer the data to an external analysis team for data analysis. Data transfer can be a sensitive as it may contain safety and efficacy data and hence, it needs to be done very carefully (refer to the **Fig – Data transfer process**).

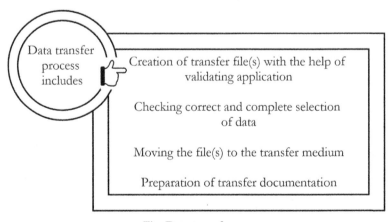

Fig: Data transfer process

Transfer metrics and transfer checklists are the tools which can be helpful for improving and documenting the whole data transfer process.

Due to the regulatory submission factor, it is imperative to maintain the audit trail of all CDM activities. It helps during regulatory audit when auditor verifies the discrepancy management process and the changes made and ensures no unauthorized changes /steps have been considered during the whole process.

Good Clinical Data Management Practices (GCDMP) guidelines provide the standards of good practice within CDM. Clinical Data Interchange Standards Consortium (CDISC), a multidisciplinary non-profit organization, has developed standards to support acquisition, exchange, submission, and archival of clinical research data and metadata (data of the data entered). It includes data regarding the individual who made the entry or a change in the clinical data, the date and time of entry/change and details of the changes that have been made.

Study Data Tabulation Model Implementation Guide for Human Clinical Trials (SDTMIG) and the Clinical Data Acquisition Standards Harmonization (CDASH) standards [available free of cost from the CDISC website (www.cdisc.org)] are two important standards. The SDTMIG standard describes the details of model and standard terminologies for the data and serves as a guide to the organization. CDASH defines the basic standards for the collection of data in a clinical trial and enlists the basic data information needed from a clinical, regulatory, and scientific perspective.

Chapter 13

AUDIT AND INSPECTION

13.1 Learnings from the chapter

- *Introduction to Audit and Inspection*

- *Importance of Audit/Inspection in clinical trial*

- *Different types of Audit and Inspection*

- *Preparation of audit/inspection*

- *Inspection process and its consequences*

13.2 Introduction

To achieve an overall efficiency and effectiveness in all the aspects of a clinical trial process, the trial processes must be audited/inspected by auditors/inspectors. Audit/Inspection verifies that the research site is functioning in a sound manner and all the processes at the investigative site are compliant with recommended standards and guidelines. It provides an insight into the seismic activities (if any) going on in the research site, which may adversely affect interest of the trial.

13.3 Audit and Inspection

Audit (Inspection) is a systematic and independent examination of trial related activities and documents to determine the following:

- whether the evaluated trial related activities were conducted and

- the data recorded, analysed and accurately reported according to the protocol, sponsor's SOP, GCP and applicable regulatory requirements

During a clinical development process, the audit can be conducted by FDA, IRB and sponsor (refer to the **Fig – Audit or inspection during clinical trial**).

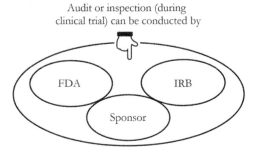

Fig: Audit or inspection during clinical trial

Audit conducted by FDA or other regulatory authority is known as "**Inspection**". Thus, Inspection can be defined as "The act by a regulatory authority(ies), of conducting an official review of documents, facilities, records, and any other resources related to the clinical trial."

13.4 Importance of Audit/Inspection

The main purpose of an audit is to determine that a clinical trial has been performed in compliance with study protocol and applicable regulatory regulations or not (refer to the **Fig – Importance of Audit/Inspection**).

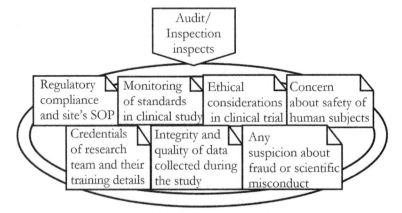

Fig: Importance of Audit/Inspection

In the process of auditing, the auditor may check the informed consent forms, the documentation of the consent process, the regulatory records, the source documents, the reported data and other trial related materials to ensure the trial is compliant.

13.5 Audit conducted by Sponsor and IRB

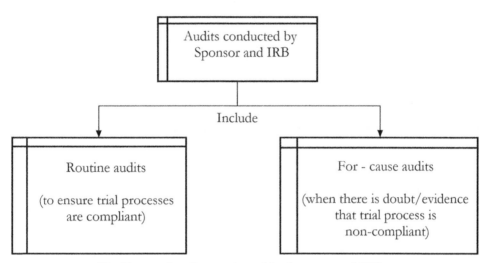

Fig: Types of audits conducted by Sponsor and IRB

Audit conducted by sponsor

13.6 Routine audits

Important features of Routine audits (which are conducted by the sponsor) have been explained in the **Fig – Routine audits**.

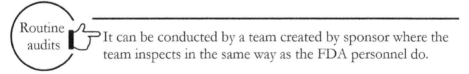

It can be conducted by a team created by sponsor where the team inspects in the same way as the FDA personnel do.

These audits ensure that the conduct of trial process is compliant with regulations and protocol and everything is in the right place in case, there is an inspection done by FDA.

During audit, if any error is found in the trial, the investigator will be instructed to correct it before visit of FDA personnel.

Fig: Routine audits

When there is multi-site trial, the sponsor estimates as to which site will be inspected and accordingly sponsor takes the audit plan.

13.7 For–cause audits

Important features of for–cause audits (which are conducted by sponsor) have been explained in the **Fig – For-cause audits**.

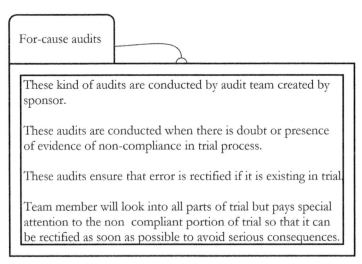

Fig: For-cause audits

13.8 Consequences of sponsor driven audit

There can be different consequences of audits which are conducted by sponsor (refer to the **Fig – Consequences of sponsor driven audit**).

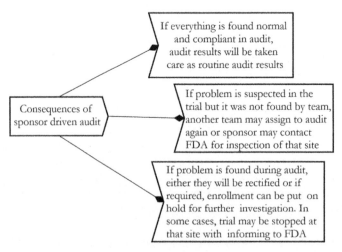

Fig: Consequences of sponsor driven audit

Audit conducted by IRB

Routine visits are held just to ensure that everything is going in accordance with compliance while for-cause audits are conducted when some problem or non- compliance is suspected at the site. It is the responsibility of IRB to inform FDA about all instances indicating harm to subjects or violence of regulations.

13.9 Inspection conducted by FDA

FDA inspects manufacturers or processors of FDA-regulated products to verify that they comply with the relevant regulations. Sponsor identifies the site (e.g. site which has recorded high enrolment) which can be inspected by the FDA and then prepares the site with the help of Clinical Research Associate (CRA) to make sure that everything is in place. This step is taken to ensure that the FDA inspectors find the site working in a correct manner by being compliant. As these inspections are important with respect to product approval, the sponsor applies the best to make a positive impression on the FDA inspectors.

13.10 Types of Inspections conducted by FDA

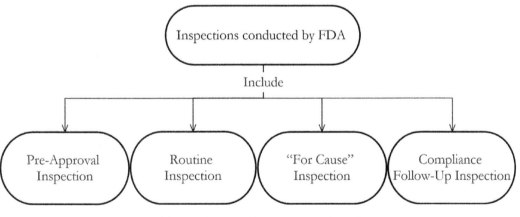

Fig: Types of inspections conducted by FDA

The different types of Inspections have been explained below:

13.11 Pre-Approval Inspection

Important features of Pre-Approval Inspection are listed in the **Fig – Pre-Approval Inspection**.

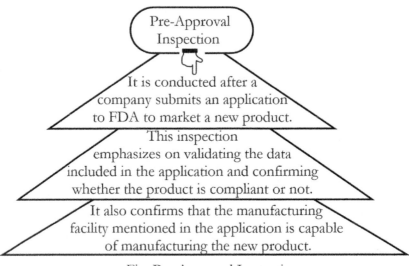

Fig: Pre-Approval Inspection

13.12 Routine Inspection

Important features of Routine Inspections are listed in the **Fig – Routine Inspections**.

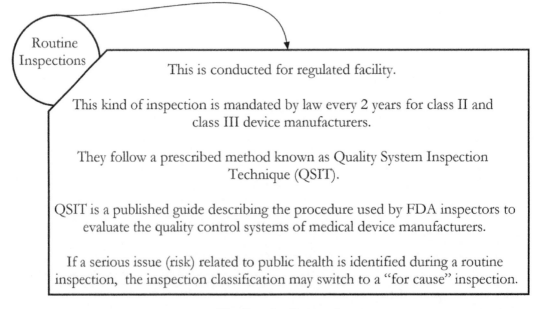

Fig: Routine Inspections

13.13 "For-cause" inspection

Important features of "For-cause" inspection is depicted in the **Fig – "For-cause" Inspection**.

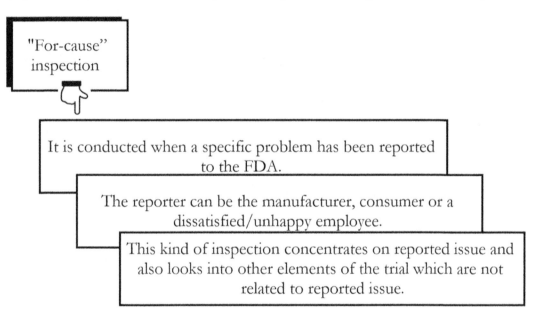

"For-cause" inspection

It is conducted when a specific problem has been reported to the FDA.

The reporter can be the manufacturer, consumer or a dissatisfied/unhappy employee.

This kind of inspection concentrates on reported issue and also looks into other elements of the trial which are not related to reported issue.

Fig: "For-cause" inspection

13.14 Compliance follow-up inspection

Important features of Compliance follow-up inspection are mentioned in the **Fig – Compliance follow-up inspection.**

It is conducted to follow up on information indicating serious problems at the research site.

It is conducted to verify that adequate corrections of previous violations are done or in order to document continuing violations to support possible regulatory actions.

Fig: Compliance follow-up inspection

13.15 Features of Audit and Inspection

Audit	Inspection
Purpose - to ensure the trial implementation and data are up to recommended standards	Purpose – to verify whether the data can be used to fully evaluate drug effects and safety, and to determine whether the drug can be allowed into the market
Usually, carried out either during or after the research	Usually, carried out after the research
Responsibility of Sponsor	Responsibility of Regulatory authority
Normally, all the trial data have not been obtained	Usually all the trial data have been obtained

13.16 Preparation for an audit/Inspection

Audit is an important aspect of a trial which assures that all the processes are being followed in a proper manner. It is important for the research team to be ready for an audit which can happen anytime during the trial and the research staff must be aware of the importance of audit and its consequences during the trial and also about the requirements of an audit process. They should get proper training on all the processes and policies related to the trial. Information about the audit date, audit location and other relevant details should be communicated to all key staff in writing and accordingly research staff need to prepare for the audit.

In the process of preparation of an audit, all research related documents such as consent forms, case report form, regulatory documents etc. should be reviewed thoroughly to present the complete and accurate documents during the audit and these documents should be easily accessible during the audit. This preparation makes the research staff ready for all the questions that might be asked by the auditors during auditing.

A room (or place) equipped with computers, telephone, internet, fax machine and other required equipment and facilities should be made ready for auditing. Research staffs must be aware of the matter that many auditors are not permitted to accept meals, so it is important to get this information in advance whether policies will allow to provide the auditors with food or not. All required records and reports should be provided to the auditors on their request.

13.17 Inspection Process

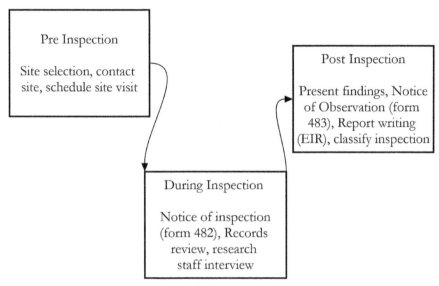

Fig: Inspection process in clinical trial

<u>Notification to the investigative site by inspector (FDA person)</u> – Research site staff will be contacted by the FDA person for deciding on a suitable time to visit. Site may get one or two weeks of time to prepare for inspection. Generally, the pre-approval and routine inspections are announced five calendar days in advance. On the other hand, the compliance follow-up inspections and "for cause" inspections are not pre-announced. FDA contacts foreign manufacturers 2 - 3 months in advance to schedule inspection.

<u>Identity proof provided by inspector at the site</u> – Inspectors need to show the investigator their credentials and a Notice of Inspections (Form 482). If they don't show these documents, it is the responsibility of investigator to check if he/she dealing with right person regarding trial matter.

<u>Availability of investigator and CRC</u> – It is compulsory for the investigator and the clinical research coordinator(CRC) to be present during the inspection. They need to provide the FDA person a good welcome at the site and also all the documents asked by inspector. All questions asked by inspector should be replied clearly by research staffs.

<u>Verification of documents</u> – Inspectors cross check all the trial processes for the conduct of trial and they also check the clinical data. They check if all documents submitted to FDA are same with the documents at the site. They can also check sponsor's records.

Review of inspection – Once audit is completed, the inspector will do a review for all the audit findings. In this review process, investigator will also be present so that he/she can clarify all the doubts asked by the inspector. In case of any significant observations, FDA Form 483 (Notice of Observation) can be issued which may describe compliance violation. FDA Form 483, includes the name of the firm and the date(s) of inspection, and list of the observations made by the inspector during the inspection.

Establishment Inspection Report (EIR) - The outcomes of the inspection are reported as No Action Indicated (NAI) or Voluntary Action Indicated (VAI) or Official Action Indicated (OAI) [refer to the **Fig – Types of outcomes of an Inspection**]. Post–audit, the FDA inspector prepares final inspection report called an "Establishment Inspection Report (EIR)".

No Action Indicated (NAI)	Voluntary Action Indicated (VAI)	Official Action Indicated (OAI)
This occurs when no objectionable conditions or practices were found during the inspection or the significance of the documented objectionable conditions found does not justify further actions.	This occurs when objectionable conditions or practices were found at research site that do not meet the threshold of regulatory significance; needed response will be specified in the letter.	This occurs when significant objectionable conditions or practices were found at the research site (worst outcome); FDA may inform IRB and sponsor for this letter and FDA may issue warning letter or may take another serious action which will be unpleasant for sponsor/investigator

Fig: Types of outcomes of an Inspection

13.18 Consequences of Inspection

There are possibilities that the sponsor may repeat the trial in case the inspection findings point towards significant problems in the trial. Study can be invalidated at that particular site in case of insufficient data or protocol violence.

Investigators can be disqualified or restricted from conducting the trial. This can add them in the "List of Disqualified and Restricted Investigators". In worst cases, the investigator may be fined and/or sentenced to prison.

Chapter 14

BIOSTATISTICS

14.1 Learnings from the chapter

- *Introduction to statistics and biostatistics*

- *Different types of data and graphical representation of data*

- *Notes on measures of data (which includes measures of central tendency, measures of dispersion and measures of shape)*

- *Concept of normal distribution and hypothesis testing*

- *Parametric and non-parametric data and their respective tests*

- *Uses of biostatistics in clinical trial*

14.2 Introduction

Biostatistics secures an important platform in the clinical research as biostatisticians play a vital role throughout the entire drug development process. They participate in many other important tasks apart from mere calculations.

14.3 Biostatistics

The term "Biostatistics" is used when statistical tools are used to the biological data (e.g., data from medicine). It covers various steps in a clinical research such as hypothesis generation, data collection, data analysis, etc. It is the science which deals with development and application of the most appropriate methods for the following processes (refer to the **Fig – Biostatistics application**)

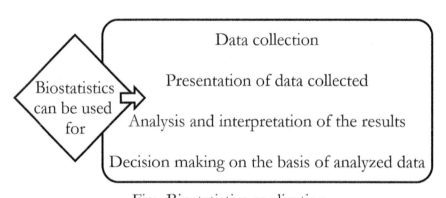

Fig: Biostatistics application

The application of statistics enables the clinical researchers to draw a reasonable and accurate inferences from gathered data/information and to make scientifically sound decisions. Proper use of statistical concepts and tools can avoid many errors/biases in clinical research.

14.4 Statistics in nutshell

Statistics deals with measured/counted facts such as height of an individual. Statistics is all about converting collected data into useful information through data collection, summarization and interpretation of collected data.

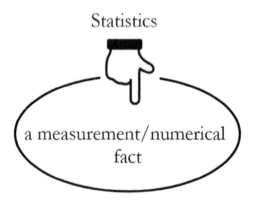

14.5 Types of Statistics

Statistics can be categorized as descriptive and inferential (refer to the **Fig – Types of Statistics**). Descriptive statistics describes (e.g., graphs) the collected data but this does not infer. On the other hand, inferential statistics concludes (makes assumptions/predictions) from the collected data.

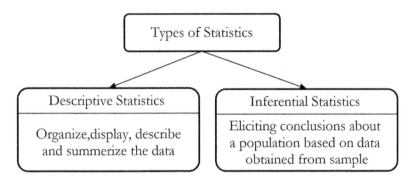

Fig: Types of Statistics

14.6 Types of data

Data is a set of values of qualitative or quantitative variables. Pieces of data are individual pieces of information. Data can exist in various forms. The different types of data are depicted in the **Fig – Types of data**.

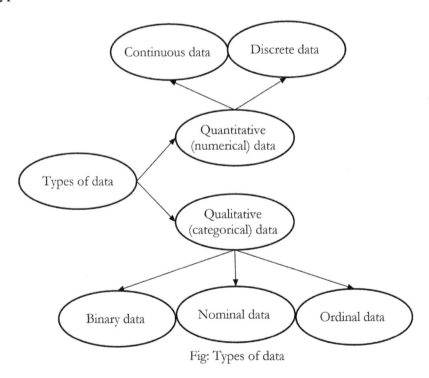

Fig: Types of data

The different types of the data have been described below:

14.7 Quantitative (numerical) data

It comprises of characteristics, which can be expressed numerically. For instance; age, weight, etc. It is of two types (refer to the **Fig – Types of Quantitative data**).

Continuous data	Discrete data
It includes any value in the given range and there is no gap in the values of the variables. It is often measured and not counted. Example - Weight of an individual	It includes only whole integer number and there are no intermediate values between each number. It is often counted and not measured. Example - Number of children in an apartment

Fig: Types of Quantitative data

14.8 Qualitative (categorical) data

It comprises of characteristics, which cannot be expressed numerically. For instance; gender, ethnicity, etc. It is of three types (refer to the **Fig – Types of Qualitative data**).

Binary data	Nominal data	Ordinal data
Variables are divided into two mutually exclusive (mutually exclusive means both events cannot occur at the same time) categories e.g., gender (binary data)-male or female (categories)	Variables are divided into more than two mutually exclusive unordered categories (categories cannot be ordered one above the another i.e. not greater or less than each other) e.g., blood groups (A, B, O, AB)	Variables are divided into more than two mutually exclusive ordered categories (categories can be ordered one above the another), e.g., grades such as mild, moderate, severe or good, average, poor

Fig: Types of Qualitative data

14.9 Graphical representation of data

Graphical representation of data helps in faster and easier interpretation of data. This method uses different types of graphs and pictorial representations of data.

14.10 Types of graphs

Different types of graphs have been explained below (refer to the **Fig – Types of graphs**).

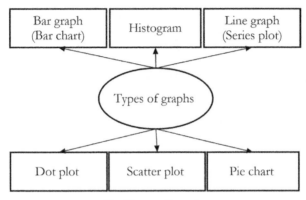

Fig: Types of graphs

14.11 Bar graph (Bar chart)

It is a kind of graph that presents grouped (categorical) data with rectangular (nonadjacent) bars with lengths proportional to the values that they represent. The bars can be plotted vertically or horizontally.

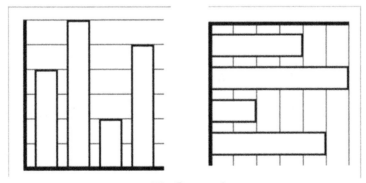

Fig: Bar graph

14.12 Histogram

This is a form of bar graph which is used for continuous class intervals. It comprises of adjacent rectangles whose area is proportional to the frequency of a variable and whose width is equal to the class interval.

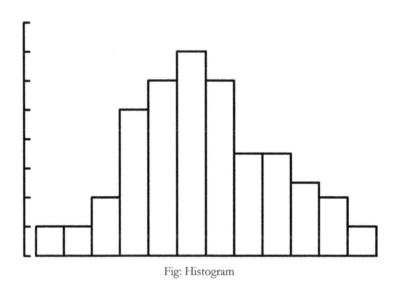

Fig: Histogram

14.13 Line graph (Series plot)

Line graphs can be used when you are plotting data that have peaks (ups) and troughs (downs). It is useful to represent trend of variables over time i.e., data that vary continuously. Usually the x-axis shows the time period and the y-axis shows what is being measured.

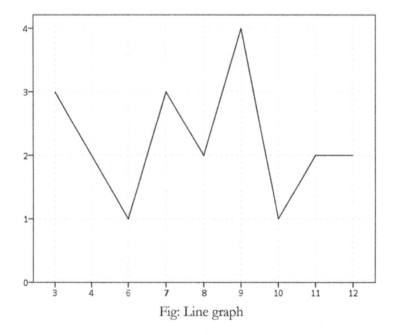

Fig: Line graph

14.14 Dot Plot

It is useful to represent a small amount of data using dots.

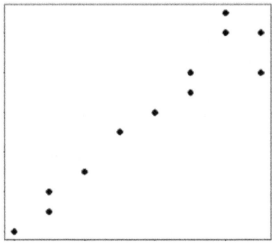

Fig: Dot plot

14.15 Scatter plot

It is used to plot data points on a horizontal and a vertical axis in the attempt to represent a relationship between two continuous variables.

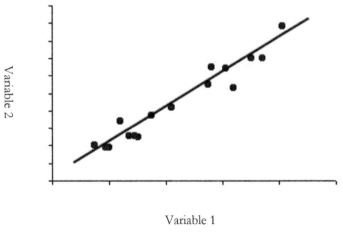

Variable 1

Fig: Scatter plot

14.16 Pie chart

This is a kind of graph in which a circle is divided into sectors and each sector represents a proportion of the whole. It is used to represent categorical data, especially data in percentage.

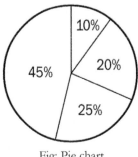

Fig: Pie chart

14.17 Measures of data

The measures of data i.e., measure of central tendency, measures of dispersion & measures of shape are explained below:

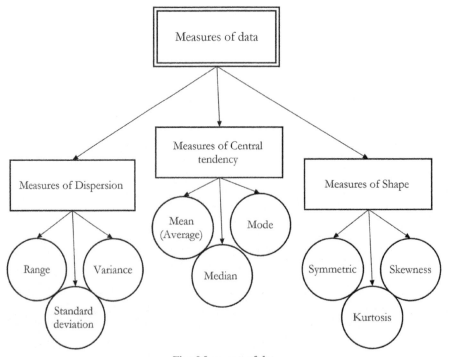

Fig:: Measures of data

14.18 Measures of Central tendency

It refers to a central or typical value for a probability distribution. It is also called a center or location of the distribution. Three important measures of central tendency are mean, median and mode (Refer to **Fig – Types of measures of Central tendency**).

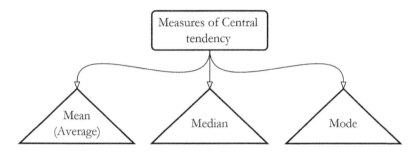

Fig: Types of Measures of Central Tendency

Types of measures of central tendency i.e., mean, median and mode have been described below:

14.19 Mean (Average)

It is denoted by "x bar". It is calculated by adding all the observations and dividing by the total number of observations.

Example – five children's history marks in 10th class are 11, 20, 11, 6,17. The mean value will be $(11+20+11+6+17)/5 = (65/5) = 13$

14.20 Median

It is the value that divides a distribution into two equal halves. In case of odd number of observations, the median is the middle value but in case of even number of observations, the median is the average of the two middle values.

Example - The median value of five children's marks (6,11,**11**,17,20) will be the middle value i.e., 11.

14.21 Mode

It is the most frequently occurring value in a set of observations.

Example - The mode value of five children's marks (6,**11,11**,17,20) will be the most frequent value i.e., 11.

14.22 Measures of Dispersion

Dispersion (also called variability, scatter, or spread) is the extent, to which a distribution is stretched or squeezed. Common examples of measures of statistical dispersion are the variance, standard deviation, and range (Refer to **Fig – Examples of Measures of Dispersion**).

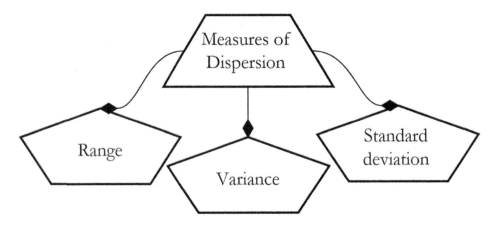

Fig: Examples of Measures of Dispersion

Measures of Dispersion i.e., range, variance and standard deviation have been explained below:

14.23 Range

It refers to the difference in values between the highest (maximum) and the lowest (minimum) observations in a given data set.

Example - five children's history marks in 10th class are 11, 20, 11, 6,17. The range value will be 20 (highest value) – 11 (lowest value) = 9

14.24 Variance

It refers to the amount of variability or spread about the mean of the sample.

Formula of variance (σ^2) – The average of the squared differences from the Mean.

The Population: divide by **N** when calculating Variance

A Sample: divide by **N-1** when calculating Variance

$$\text{Variance (Population)} \quad \sigma^2 = \frac{\sum (X - \mu)^2}{N}$$

$$\text{Variance (Sample)} \quad s^2 = \frac{\sum (X - \bar{X})^2}{n-1}$$

Where;
N or n- total number of data values
X - individual data value
μ or $\bar{X}$ - mean

14.25 Standard deviation

The standard deviation (σ) is the square root of the variance.

Formulas of standard deviation:

$$\text{Standard deviation (Population)} \quad \sigma = \sqrt{\frac{\sum (x - \mu)^2}{N}}$$

$$\text{Standard deviation (Sample)} \quad s = \sqrt{\frac{\sum (x - \bar{x})^2}{n-1}}$$

Where;
N or n- total number of data values
X - individual data value
μ or $\bar{x}$ - mean

The variance and the standard deviation give us a numerical measure of the scatter of a data set. These measures are useful for making comparisons between data sets that go beyond simple visual impressions.

14.26 Standard Error of Mean

Standard Error of Mean

In statistics, a sample mean deviates from the actual mean of a population; this deviation is the standard error. The standard error of the mean gives an estimate of the degree to which the sample mean(x) varies from the population mean (μ). This measure is used to calculate confidence interval(CI). A confidence interval is the probability that a value will fall between an upper and lower bound of a probability distribution.

Standard deviation is used to describe data where as standard error (or confidence interval) is used to describe the outcome of a study.

Standard Error = standard deviation of sample mean/square root of sample size

14.27 Measures of Shape

It describes the distribution (or pattern) of the data within a dataset. Measure of shape for quantitative data is possible because there is a logical order to the values, and the 'low' and 'high' end values on the x-axis can be identified. But, measure of shape for a qualitative data is not possible because data are not numeric.

Three types of shapes (refer to the **Fig – Types of shapes**) have been explained below:

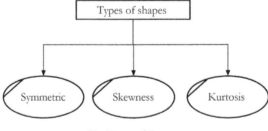

Fig: Types of shapes

14.28 Symmetric

Distributions that have the same shape on both sides of the centre are called symmetric. A symmetric distribution with only one peak is known as "normal distribution".

14.29 Skewness

Skewness measures the extent (degree) of asymmetry in a distribution (refer to the **Fig – Skewness**). Skewness is the tendency for the values to be more frequent around the high or low ends of the x-axis.

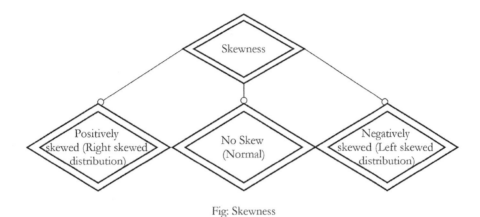

Fig: Skewness

Different forms of skewness i.e., positively skewed and negatively skewed have been described below:

14.30 Positively skewed (Right – skewed distribution)

A distribution is said to be positively skewed when the tail on the right side of the histogram is longer than the left side. Most of the values tend to cluster toward the left side of the x-axis with increasingly fewer values at the right side of the x-axis (refer to the **Fig – Positively skewed**).

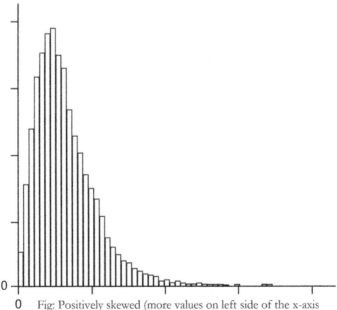

Fig: Positively skewed (more values on left side of the x-axis with increasingly fewer values at the right side of the x-axis)

14.31 Negatively skewed (Left - skewed distribution)

A distribution is said to be negatively skewed when the tail on the left side of the histogram is longer than the right side. Most of the values tend to cluster toward the right side of the x-axis (i.e. the larger values), with increasingly less values on the left side of the x-axis (i.e. the smaller values) [refer to the **Fig – Negatively skewed**]

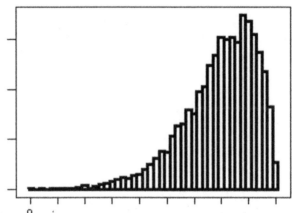

Fig: Negatively skewed (more values on right side of the x-axis
with increasingly less values on the left side of the x-axis)

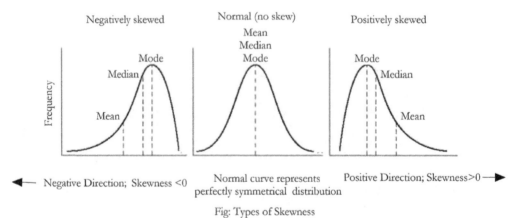

Fig: Types of Skewness

14.32 Kurtosis (Mesokurtic, Leptokurtic & Platykurtic)

Kurtosis is the measure of the thickness or heaviness of the tails of a distribution. Kurtosis is a measure of whether the data are heavy-tailed or light-tailed relative to a normal distribution. Mesokurtic, Leptokurtic and Platykurtic are different types of Kurtosis (refer to the **Fig – Types of Kurtosis & Fig – Kurtosis).**

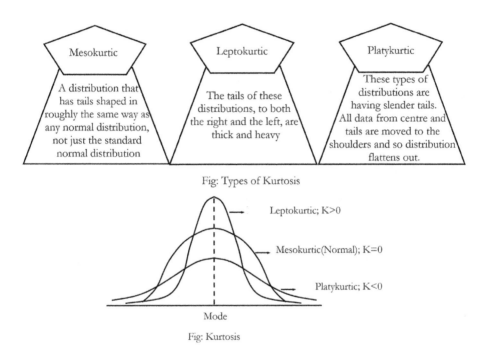

Fig: Types of Kurtosis

Fig: Kurtosis

14.33 Normal Distribution

Normal distribution details about the extent of normal biological variation that exists with respect to the given biological variable. It constitutes a group of curves defined uniquely by two parameters i.e., mean (forms the centre of the curve) and standard deviation (forms the extent of scatter around mean). The normal distribution is sometimes informally called the bell curve.

14.34 Properties of Normal Distribution

The important properties of normal distribution are listed in the **Fig – Properties of Normal distribution.**

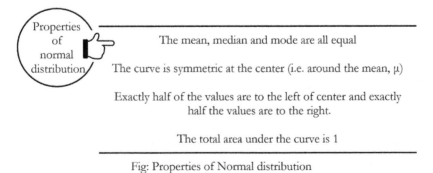

Fig: Properties of Normal distribution

Data can be spread out in different ways such as more data on left, more data on right or simply jumbled up. But, then again data also tends to accumulate around the central value and forms normal distribution.

Most of the values are clustered near the mean and a few values are near the tails. The standard deviation controls the spread of the distribution. A smaller standard deviation means that the data is tightly clustered around the mean; the normal distribution will be taller. A larger standard deviation means that the data is spread out around the mean; the normal distribution will be flatter and wider.

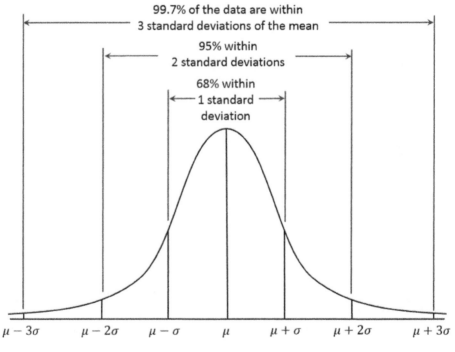

Fig: Normal distribution

Typically, if observations fall under normal distribution curve, then mean ± 1SD (standard deviation) cover about 68% of the observations, mean ±2 SD cover about 95% of the observations and mean ±3SD cover about 99.7% of the total observations.

14.35 Types of test data and their respective statistical tests

It is not possible to collect the data on individual basis (in a population of interest). Hence, the sample (representative of population of interest) is analysed through utilization of statistical methods. Sample gives an overall estimation for a population. Statistics calculates parameters such as mean, standard deviation and other parameters for sample.

To work with data in statistics, it is important to understand the kind of test data i.e., parametric or non-parametric data (refer to the **Fig – Kinds of test data**).

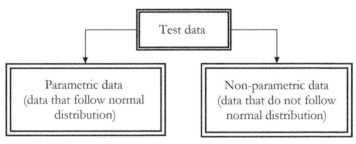

Fig: Kinds of test data

Test of significance applicable to parametric data and non-parametric data are different. Parametric statistical tests depend on assumptions about the shape of the distribution (i.e., assume a normal distribution) in the underlying population and about the parameters (i.e., means and standard deviations) of the assumed distribution. Nonparametric statistical tests depend on few assumptions or no assumptions about the shape or parameters of the population distribution from which the sample is taken.

14.36 Features of Parametric and Non-parametric tests

Parametric test	Non-parametric test
Population information - totally known	Population information – not available
Specific assumption about the population	No specific assumption about the population
Null hypothesis construction – based on parameters of population distribution	Null hypothesis construction – free from parameters
Tests are based on population distribution and applicable to variables only	Tests are arbitrary and applicable to both variables and attributes
Most appropriate for ratio data (e.g., age) and interval data (e.g., measure of temperature)	Most appropriate for ordinal data (e.g., education) and nominal data (e.g., gender); although limited use for ratio and interval data
Powerful test (if exists)	Less powerful test (because uses less information)

14.37 Which test to use – Parametric or Non-parametric test

There can be different bases for the selection of the type of test (Parametric/Non-Parametric) which can be used for analysis purpose (refer to the **Fig – Selection parameters – Parametric and Non-parametric test**).

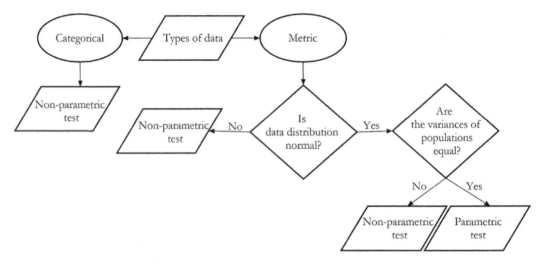

Fig:: Selection parameters - Parametric and Non-parametric test

14.38 Examples of Parametric and Non-Parametric tests (depending on the purpose of analysis)

Few Examples regarding Parametric and Non-Parametric tests (depending on the purpose of analysis) are listed in the below table:

Purpose	Parametric test	Non-parametric test
Comparison of several groups	ANOVA	Kruskal-Wallis test
Comparison of two independent groups	t-test for independent samples	Wilcoxon rank sum test
Test the difference between paired observation	t-test for paired observation	Wilcoxon signed – rank test
Test the association between two qualitative variables	–	Chi-square test

14.39 Statistical packages – examples

• Microsoft Excel - Software developed and manufactured by Microsoft Corporation that allows users to organize, format, and calculate data with formulas using a spreadsheet system broken up by rows and columns.

• SPSS - The software name originally stood for Statistical Package for the Social Sciences (SPSS) reflecting the original market, although the software is now popular in other fields as well, including the health sciences and marketing.

• SAS – SAS (Statistical Analysis System) is a software suite that can mine, alter, manage and retrieve data from a variety of sources and perform statistical analysis on it.

14.40 Use of Biostatistics in Clinical trial

Clinical trial always works to check the probability of happenings. For example, probability of a drug to bind to a particular receptor at target site. That means, a drug may or may not bind to the site. Biostatistics helps researcher to make a strongest possible conclusion from the limited amount of biological data. Thus, the most important time to involve a biostatistician is at the beginning of the trial. This allows the biostatistician to understand the design of the study and thus to provide inputs on hypothesis testing and analysis and so on (refer to the **Fig – Biostatistics -basic functions**).

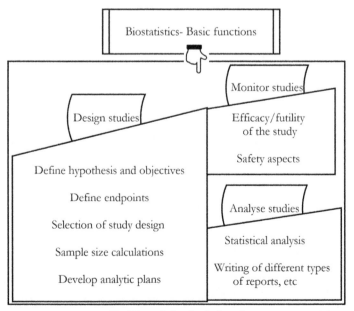

Fig: Biostatistics- basic functions

In the early part of the trial, the biostatisticians get involved in defining the study objectives, the study designs and the statistical methods that can be used to get correct clinical inferences. They also work on defining the endpoints, the sample size, the interim analysis plans and the required procedures.

14.41 Use of biostatistics in calculating the sample size

Estimation of appropriate sample size is an important factor for establishing significant results within the defined timeline. Hence, correct calculation of sample size (refer to the **Fig – Calculation of sample size**) is a critical step. A wrong sample size may lead to invalid result and also to waste of resources, time and energy. Hence, appropriate sample size is important for eliciting significant output in a set timeline which can be done with the help of an efficient biostatician.

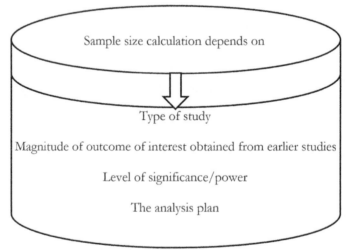

Fig: Calculation of sample size

14.42 Use of biostatistics in calculating Endpoint - examples

- Mean and mode can be useful to calculate the quantitative (continuous) measurement which represents a specific count such as blood pressure, weight.

- Odd ratio and risk ratio can be helpful to calculate the binary measurement which represents whether an incidence has taken place such as death from any reason.

14.43 Endpoints

The endpoint of a clinical trial is a pre-defined event. For example, the occurrence of a disease, the occurrence of a symptom, or a particular laboratory result. Once someone reaches the endpoint, they are generally excluded from further research in the trial.

The endpoints (or outcomes), determined for each study participant, are the quantitative measurements required by the objectives. The endpoints of a clinical trial are usually included in the study objectives.

14.44 Types of Endpoints

Endpoints can be primary and secondary. In some cases, they can be replaced by surrogate endpoints (refer to **Fig – Types of Endpoints**). Endpoints help in deciding whether to accept or reject null hypothesis.

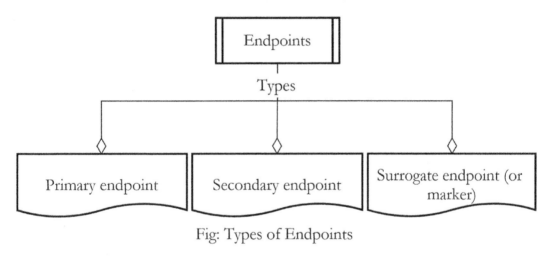

Fig: Types of Endpoints

Types of Endpoints have been explained below:

14.45 Primary endpoint

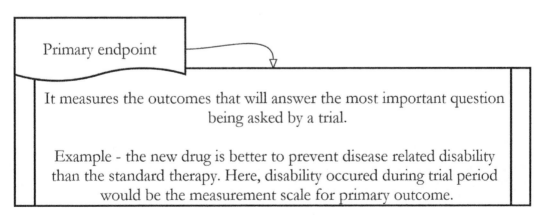

14.46 Secondary endpoint

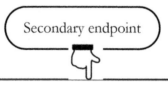

It determines the other relevant questions about the same study.

Example - if there is reduction in the disease measures other than disability
(Here, disability is primary outcome).

14.47 Surrogate endpoint (or Marker)

It is a laboratory or physical measurement used in clinical trials to indicate the
effect of a certain treatment and can be used in a place of a clinical endpoint,
which is usually acceptable as evidence of efficacy for the regulatory purposes.

The National Institutes of Health(USA) defines surrogate endpoint as "a
biomarker intended to substitute for a clinical endpoint". Surrogate markers are
used when the primary endpoint is undesired (e.g., death), or when the number
of events is very small, thus making it impractical to conduct a clinical trial to
gather a statistically significant number of endpoints.

Example
High cholesterol levels may or may not increase the chance of heart disease
in people. On the other hand, some people with normal cholesterol levels
may suffer from heart disease. Dying due to heart disease is the clinical
endpoint but cholesterol is a surrogate endpoint. Here, in trial a specific drug
can be proved effective in reducing cholesterol without showing directly
that it prevents death.

Biostaticians may also get involved in the interim analysis plan to assess the safety and efficacy of
the investigational product during the development process. In this process, the biostatistician
of research team and an independent statistician together can conduct analysis for an unbiased

result. During manuscript/reports writing at the end of trial, the biostatician may need to do the following:

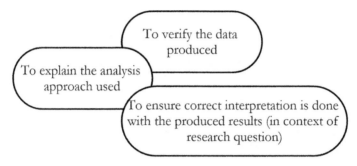

14.48 Hypothesis testing

Hypothesis testing is a kind of statistical inference that can be used to draw conclusions from a sample population about a population probability distribution.

(A probability distribution describes how the values of a random variable is distributed. A random variable is a numerical characteristic of each event in a sample space, or equivalently, each individual in a population. Example of random variable- Heights of individuals in a large population).

An observed difference or association between two groups or variables can be a real difference or can be due to mere chance. Researcher tries to determine this difference between two groups or the association between two variables. Hypothesis testing helps to find out the observed difference/association is due to chance or not (refer to the **Fig – Hypothesis assumptions**).

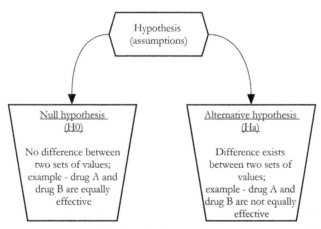

Fig: Hypothesis assumptions

14.49 Null hypothesis and Alternative (Researcher) hypothesis

Null hypothesis is established with an aim to be accepted or rejected in order to support an alternative (researcher) hypothesis. Most often, the null hypothesis refers to an existing or previous evidence which is just opposite to alternative hypothesis, which represents what researcher actually assumes the reason (cause) for a phenomenon. Null hypothesis will be considered true till the alternative hypothesis is not proved true with the help of statistical evidences. Hence, it is a must that the null hypothesis and the alternative hypothesis should be mutually exclusive and exhaustive.

14.50 Steps in Hypothesis Testing

Fig – Hypothesis testing - steps is a summarized depiction of the process of hypothesis testing. The process of hypothesis testing has been explained below:

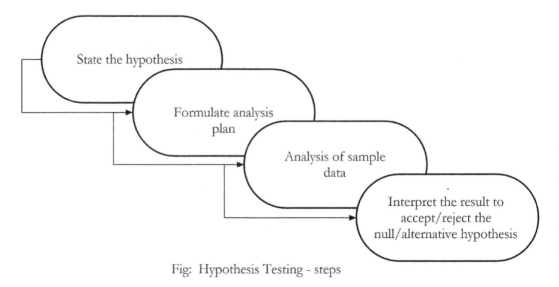

Fig: Hypothesis Testing - steps

1.   State the hypothesis assumptions - Null Hypothesis and Alternative Hypothesis

2.   Formulate an analysis plan – which includes the following:

2.1   Selection of significance level (α) – the criterion used for rejecting the null hypothesis; it should be set before testing the null hypothesis.

    ✓   The first step is to find out the difference between the results of the experiment and the null hypothesis. Then, assuming that the null hypothesis is true, the probability of a difference that large (or larger) is computed. The final step is to compare this probability to the significance level.

✓ If the probability is less than or equal to the significance level, then the null hypothesis is rejected and the outcome is said to be "statistically significant" (**means probably true** not due to chance).

Most often, the experimenters have used either the 0.05 level (5% level or 1 in 20) or the 0.01 level (1% level or 1 in 100), although the choice of levels is largely subjective. 5% significant level means researcher is ready to take 5 percent chance of wrong result. In the same way, 1% significant level means researcher is expecting to be 99% sure about his/her alternative hypothesis.

2.2 Choosing a test statistic and compute p-value – test statistics is calculated from sample data to determine the acceptance/rejection of null hypothesis. There are various tests such as t-test, z-test for continuous data, chi-square test for proportions, etc. With the help of t-test, "p-value (probability of occurrence of an event)" can be derived.

3. Analysis of sample data – p-value provides a convenient basis for eliciting conclusions in hypothesis testing. It measures how compatible the sample results are with the null hypothesis.

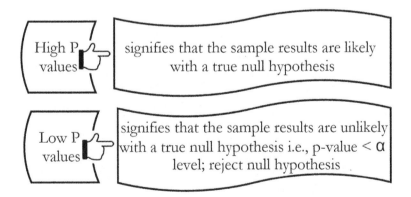

High P values ☞ signifies that the sample results are likely with a true null hypothesis

Low P values ☞ signifies that the sample results are unlikely with a true null hypothesis i.e., p-value < α level; reject null hypothesis

Low p-value suggests that the researcher sample provides enough evidence that he/she can reject the null hypothesis for the whole population. P value is the probability of obtaining a result at least as extreme as that observed in a study by chance alone, assuming that the null hypothesis is true. The final decision to accept or reject the null hypothesis depends on p-value.

14.51 Kinds of errors

Hypothesis testing is based on sample data hence, chances of errors must be considered. There are two kinds of errors that can be made in significance testing (refer to the **Fig – Kinds of errors during significance testing**).

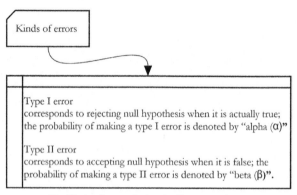

Fig: Kinds of errors during significance testing

The probability of committing a type I error is equal to the level of significance that was set for the hypothesis test. Therefore, if the level of significance is 0.05, there is a 5% chance a type I error may occur. The probability of committing a type II error is dependent on the power of the test. The power of test can be increased by increasing the sample size, which decreases the risk of committing a type II error.

Example for Type I and Type II error

Suppose a pharmaceutical firm decides to test and compare how effective two of its drugs are for treating hypertension.

The hypothesis assumptions taken in this research are as follows:

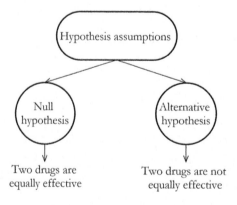

The firm conducts a clinical trial for 1,000 patients with hypertension to compare both the drugs. The firm plans to expose an equal number of patients to both drugs to study the hypothesis assumptions. Significance level is set to 0.05, which indicates that firm is willing to accept a 5% chance it may reject the null hypothesis when it is true (5% chance of committing a type I error). Now suppose the beta is calculated to be 0.035 (3.5%); this means that the probability of committing a type II error is 3.5%. If the two medications are not equal, the null hypothesis should be rejected but if the firm does not reject the null hypothesis when the drugs are not equally effective, a type II error occurs.

4. Interpret the result to accept/reject the null/alternative hypothesis – if the sample results are unlikely to the stated null hypothesis, researcher will reject the null hypothesis and this is done through comparing p-value with the significance level. If p-value comes lesser than significance level, null hypothesis will be rejected.

Chapter 15

MEDICAL WRITING

15.1 Learnings from the chapter

• *Introduction to medical writing with its scope and importance in clinical research*

• *Different types of medical writing and importance of quality in writings*

• *Characteristics of medical writers and their different roles in a clinical research (trial)*

• *Brief notes on different regulatory documents such as IB, INDA, NDA, PMA, BLA, PSUR, DSUR, etc.*

15.2 Introduction

Medical writing is an indispensable activity in clinical research and it is required at every stage of developing a therapeutic product. It communicates complex information in a clear, concise, credible and complete form. Medical writing is also known as medical communications, scientific writing, and scientific communications. Regulatory authorities prefer to accept the document which is precise and according to the required format. They study the submitted documents (by drug developers) thoroughly to check the accuracy of submitted document.

15.3 Medical writing

Medical writing is both a science and an art. It requires an understanding in medical science and an aptitude for writing. In addition, being up to date with the relevant guidelines and possessing a thorough knowledge of specific requirements for different types of medical documents is a must.

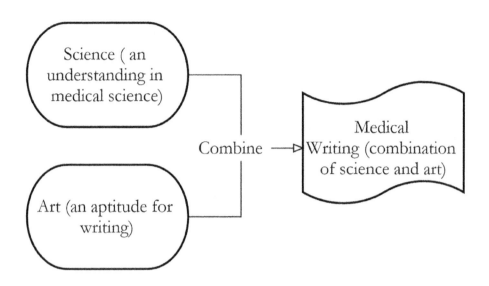

15.4 Importance of Medical writing

In the pharmaceutical world, the drug developers realized that it is important to have a separate department to create well-structured documents related to clinical trial activities. As it is known to all that clinical trials are highly regulatory and scientifically oriented process. Hence, it demands for well written, standards compliant documents that will be easily understandable to target audiences such as regulators, public, etc.

Looking into the history, Hippocrates "Father of Medicine" suggested that doctors while treating their patients should always follow a systemic way of observing and recording. This process would enable them to understand the natural history of the illness which in-turn would help forecasting the development of the illness in future. He created documentations about different medical conditions such as hemorrhoids, surgery, fractures, ulcers, sacred disease (one of the first recorded observations of epilepsy in humans) and also the book of Aphorisms. In the same way, Andreas Vesalius "Father of Anatomy", created drawings of the human body that greatly advanced the study of anatomy.

Thus, medical writing plays an important role in the life of any medicinal product. Some of the important roles are listed in the **Fig – Importance of Medical writing.**

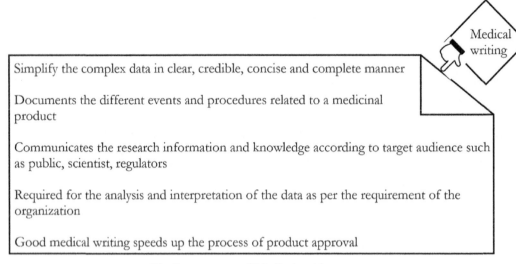

Fig: Importance of Medical writing

15.5 Scope of Medical writing

Medical writing carries the possibility of working in various fields of writing such as the field related to research, the field related to regulation, the field related to general public from the drug/medical information standpoint, the field related to healthcare professionals, the field related to academics and so on. Hence, medical writing covers variety of fields, some of which are mentioned in the **Fig – Scope of Medical writing**.

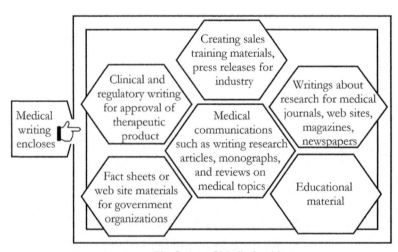

Fig: Scope of Medical writing

15.6 Types of medical writing

During the research, medical writers work closely with the professionals in the biostatistical, pharmacovigilance, project management, clinical data management, quality assurance, quality control teams to deliver accurate, timely and cost-effective documents to the highest ethical and scientific standards. Post research, writers provides assistance in developing documents on the need basis such as writing for physician, public, pharma company, etc. Thus, medical writing can be used on the requirements of general population, healthcare field, regulatory field, etc. The classification of these various types of writings are shown in the **Fig – Types of medical writing.**

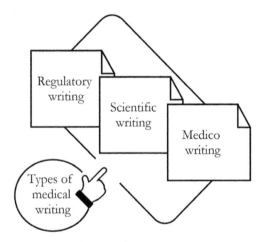

Fig: Types of Medical writing

The types of medical writing have been explained below:

15.7 Regulatory writing

This type of writing involves production of regulatory documents (usually required for regulatory purposes). These documents should be written in accordance with relevant guidance enclosing clear explanation of the information to the target audience.

15.8 Scientific writing

This type of writing requires an ability to understand the data and writing those data in a non-promotional and unbiased form. Scientific writing is scientific and evidence based in nature.

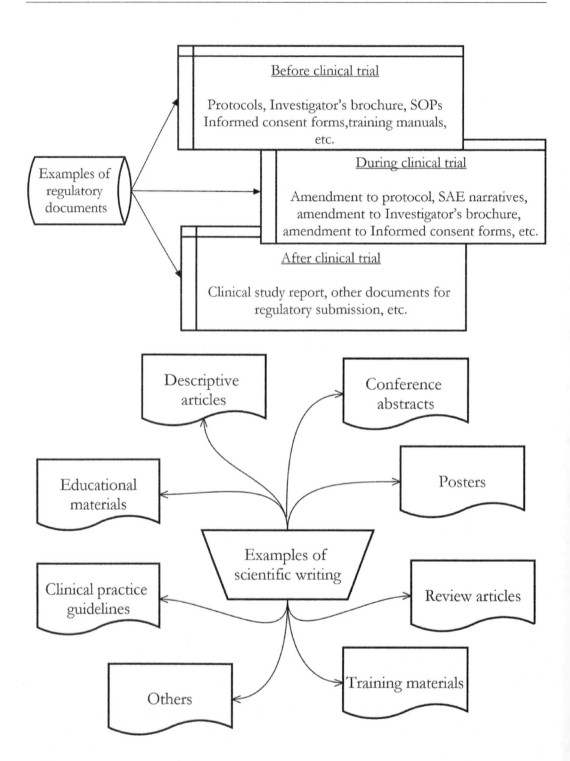

15.9 Medico writing

This type of writing seeks writers who have a rhetoric ability to balance science and business to write data in promotional form. Medico writing is also scientific and evidence based in nature.

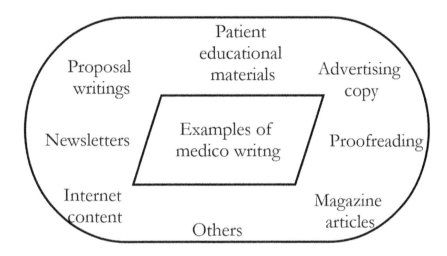

15.10 Medical Writer

Medical writing is the activity of producing scientific documentation by a specialized writer called "Medical Writer" who is generally not one of the scientists or doctors who performed the research.

15.11 Qualities of good Medical writer

To become a good medical writer, it is a must to have a clear understanding of medical concepts and regulatory guidelines along with flawless writing skills. Likewise, some other qualities of a good medical writer are capsuled in the **Fig – Qualities of good medical writer.**

15.12 Important roles of Medical writer

Medical writers contribute in different kinds of writing whether it is before approval or post approval of a medicinal product. Some important roles of medical writers are depicted in the **Fig – Important roles of Medical writer.**

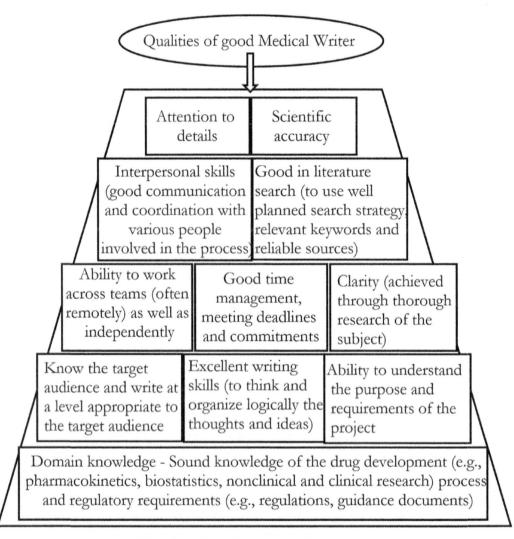

Fig: Qualities of good medical writer

15.13 Documents generated by the medical writers during a clinical trial

During a clinical trial, a number of clinical documents are produced by medical writers. The success of a trial depends on the proper handling of these documents at the investigative site and the sponsor site. These documents are required during audit /inspection which assures the validity of the trial conduct and the integrity of data collected. The various documents produced during a clinical trial are depicted in the **Fig – Documents generated during clinical trial**.

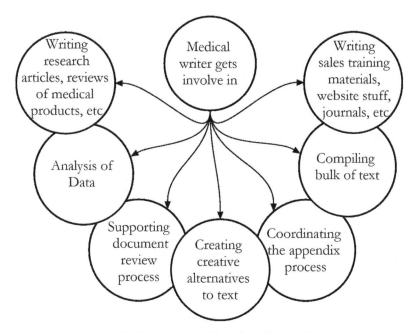

Fig: Important roles of medical writers

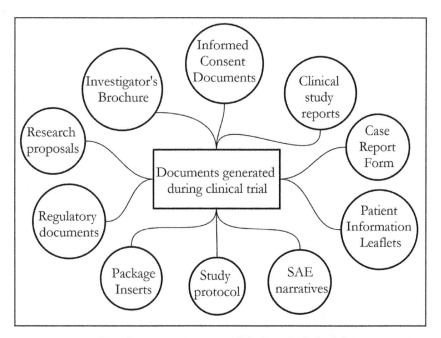

Fig: Documents generated during clinical trial

These documents are useful in demonstrating the compliance maintained by the investigator, sponsor and monitor with standards of Good Clinical Practice and with all applicable regulatory requirements.

15.14 Importance of quality in document writing

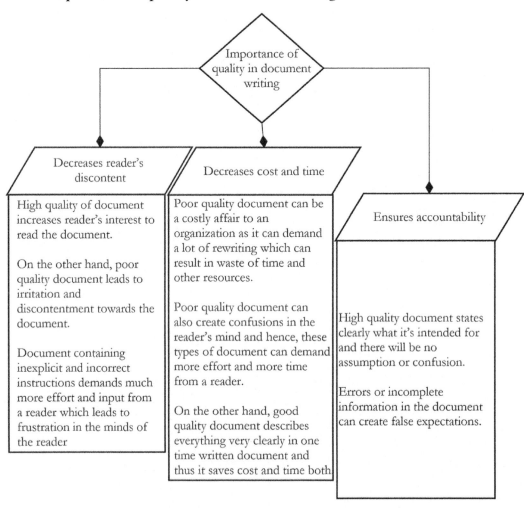

15.15 Regulations and medical writing

Different regulatory agencies (e.g., FDA, EU, CDSCO, etc.) of different countries have their own specific regulations along with some international common set guidelines. These regulations and guidelines provide guidance for writing different specific documents required in the life of medicinal product. Medical writing involves writing different kinds of scientific documents such as research related, regulatory related, drug and disease related, publication related. Hence, medical writers must be thorough with the relevant regulations and guidelines when preparing a specific document for regulatory submission.

15.16 Some important documents – Short introduction

15.17 Investigator Brochure (IB)

The Investigator brochure is a compilation of clinical and non-clinical data on the investigational product(s) that are relevant to the study of the product(s) in human subjects. The IB is a document of critical importance throughout the drug development process and is updated with new information as it becomes available. The sponsor is responsible for keeping the information in the IB up-to-date.

IB provides:

- The investigator and other research staffs with background information about the investigational product in order to help them work in line with the study protocol

- Information which is helpful in assessing the appropriateness of a trial, including the benefit-risk ratio, in an independent and unbiased way

- Insight supporting the clinical management of study participants during the clinical trial, including information about doses, dose frequency, methods of administration, and safety monitoring procedures.

15.18 Clinical Study Report (CSR)

A CSR is a scientific document addressing efficacy and safety of a trial product. It is not a sales or marketing tool. Its content is similar to that of a peer-reviewed academic paper. CSR provides detailed information about the methods and results of a clinical trial.

According to the ICH Guideline E3, a CSR is an integrated report of a study of any therapeutic, prophylactic or diagnostic agent in which the clinical and statistical description, presentations and analyses are provided in a single report, incorporating tables and figures into the main text of the report and in appendices.

15.19 Investigational New Drug Application (INDA)

Once the drug developer has established through animal studies that the investigational drug is reasonably safe for initial use in humans, and that it shows sufficient promise as a treatment to justify commercial development, INDA needs to be submitted to the FDA by drug developers for getting permission to conduct further steps i.e., transition to clinical studies from pre-clinical studies. The authority (FDA) will review the application and concludes whether to permit clinical trial or not for that particular investigational product.

15.20 Investigational Device Exemption (IDE)

An investigational Device Exemption (IDE) is an application which allows the investigational device (a medical device which is the subject of a clinical study) to be used in a clinical study in order to collect and evaluate the efficacy and/or safety of the investigational device. Clinical investigations undertaken to develop safety and efficacy data for medical devices must be conducted according to the requirements of the Investigational Device Exemption (IDE) regulations (with some exceptions).

15.21 Biologics License Application (BLA)

A biologics license application (BLA) generally applies to vaccines and other allergenic drug products, blood products, and cellular and genetic therapies. Granting of the license certifies that biological product is safe, pure, and potent, and that the facility in which it is manufactured meets standards designed to ensure that it continues to be safe, pure, and potent. A BLA is submitted after an investigational new drug has been approved.

15.22 Premarket approval (PMA)

Premarket approval (PMA) is the FDA process of scientific and regulatory review to evaluate the safety and effectiveness of Class III medical devices. Class III devices are those which support or sustain human life. These devices are of substantial importance in preventing impairment of human health or which present a potential, unreasonable risk of illness or injury; e.g., implantable pacemakers, breast implants. PMA is the most stringent type of device marketing application required by the FDA. To gain approval, the manufacturer must present adequate scientific evidence to assure that the device is safe and effective for its intended use(s). This standard is higher than is required for 510(k) submissions.

15.23 Premarket Notification (510(k))

A 510(k) is a premarket submission made to FDA to demonstrate that the device to be marketed is at least as safe and effective, i.e., substantially equivalent, to a legally marketed device which is not subject to PMA. Submission of 510(k) to the FDA is must when manufacture wants to introduce following in US market:

- Class II medical devices (devices that pose a moderate level of risk to the user; e.g., intravenous administration sets, sutures,)

- Small number of Class I device (simple devices with minimal risk to the user; e.g., enemas, elastic bandages) and class III device (devices that pose a serious level of risk to the user; e.g., implantable pacemakers, breast implants.)

- IVDs (In vitro diagnostic medical devices)

- Change in the intended use of their medical device

- Change in the technology of a cleared device in such a way that it may significantly affect the device's safety or effectiveness

The FDA does not "approve" 510(k) submissions. It "clears" them. It is not legal to advertise a 510(k)-cleared device as "FDA-approved."

15.24 New Drug Application (NDA)

When the sponsor of a new drug believes that enough evidence on the drug's safety and effectiveness has been obtained to meet FDA's requirements for marketing approval, the sponsor submits to FDA a new drug application (NDA). The application must contain data from specific technical viewpoints for review, including chemistry, pharmacology, medical, biopharmaceutics, and statistics. If the NDA is approved, the product can be introduced to the general population.

15.25 Abbreviated New Drug Application (ANDA)

Generic drug applications are called "abbreviated" because they are not required to include preclinical (animal) and clinical (human) data to establish safety and efficacy of the candidate product. However, a generic applicant must scientifically demonstrate that its product is bioequivalent to the original product (i.e., performs in the same manner as the original drug). Once approved, an applicant may manufacture and market the generic drug product to provide a safe, effective, low cost alternative to the public. A generic drug product is one that is comparable to an innovator drug product in dosage form, strength, route of administration, quality, performance characteristics & intended use. The FDA will not approve the generic unless it is equally safe and effective.

15.26 Supplemental New Drug Application (sNDA)/ supplemental biologics license application (sBLA)

To add a new change/indication to the labeling of an approved drug, a sponsor must obtain approval of a supplemental new drug application (sNDA) or supplemental biologics license application (sBLA). It is an application that when approved will allow a company to make changes in a product that already has an approved NDA.

15.27 Periodic Safety Update Report (PSUR)/Periodic Benefit Risk Evaluation Report (PBRER)

A Periodic Safety Update Report (PSUR) is a pharmacovigilance document intended to provide an update of the worldwide safety experience of a medicinal product to regulatory authorities at defined time points post-authorization.

The PSUR has got a new identity with a new name the 'Periodic Benefit Risk Evaluation Report' or 'PBRER', (pronounced pee-brer).

A PBRER is intended to present a periodic, comprehensive, concise and critical analysis of new or emerging information on the risks of the health product, and on its benefits in approved indications, to enable an appraisal of the product's overall benefit-risk profile.

This new concept represents an evolution of the traditional Periodic Safety Update Report (PSUR) from an interval safety report to a cumulative benefit-risk report. The "new" PSUR will evaluate not just the safety aspects of the drug the way the old PSUR did, but it will now evaluate the benefits of the drug. The benefits and risks will be weighed in the document and a benefit/risk (BR) evaluation will be made. It has changed the focus from individual case safety reports to aggregate data evaluation. In addition, the broadened scope of PBRER increased the need for integrating information within the report.

15.28 Development Safety Update Report (DSUR)

The DSUR is the pre-marketing report equivalent to the post-marketing Periodic Safety Update Report (PSUR). It is a stand-alone document which can be referred for analysis purpose. The purpose of a DSUR is to present a comprehensive, scientific annual review and evaluation of pertinent safety information collected during the reporting period related to a drug under investigation, whether or not it is marketed. It also notes actions taken to reflect new or ongoing risks. The document is submitted to regulatory authorities and sometimes also to Ethics Committees/IRBs.

Chapter 16

PHARMACOLOGY (SNAPSHOT)

16.1 Learnings from the chapter

- *Introduction to pharmacology and overview of drug life in human body*
- *Pharmacokinetics and pharmacodynamics*
- *Routes of drug administration*
- *Drug definition and drug nomenclature with few examples*

16.2 Introduction

Drug is a substance which is expected to give therapeutic responses when administered in a living system. A drug can be administered through different routes in different forms. To show the effect in a living body, the drug undergoes many changes inside body which is needed to be studied for estimating the drug action in a living system and vice versa.

16.3 Pharmacology

Pharmacology is the branch of medicine concerned with the uses, effects and modes of action of drugs. In simple words, pharmacology studies drugs and their interaction with the living body. Two main areas of pharmacology are pharmacodynamics and pharmacokinetics (refer to the **Fig – Pharmacology**).

16.4 Overview of drug life inside a human body

When a drug enters a human body, it passes though many events. These various events can be placed in two branches i.e., Pharmacokinetics (PK) and pharmacodynamics (PD) (refer to the **Fig – Pharmacokinetics & Pharmacodynamics**).

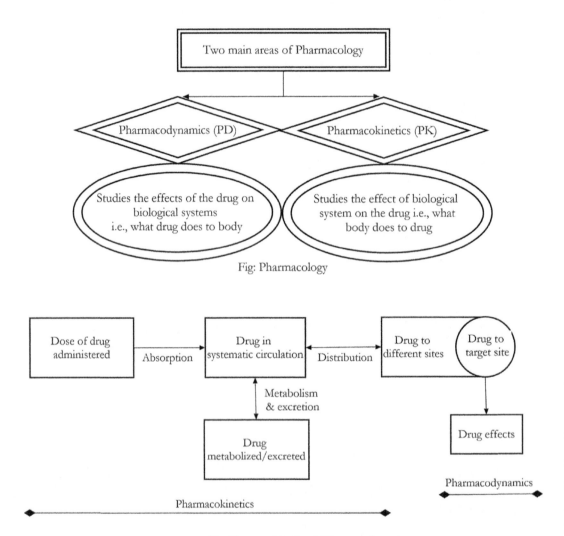

Fig: Pharmacology

Fig: Pharmacokinetics & Pharmacodynamics

16.5 Pharmacodynamics

Pharmacodynamics is the study of how a drug acts on a living body. It specifies the biological (pharmacological, physiological, biochemical and toxic) response and the duration and magnitude of response observed relative to the concentration of drug at an active site in the organism. The drug concentration level in plasma and urine in the body system are important measures to check efficacy of administered drug.

Along with therapeutic effect, drug carries some toxic effects as well (refer to the **Fig – Pharmacodynamics**).

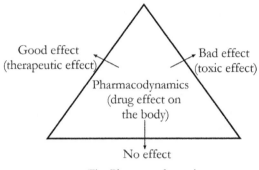

Fig: Pharmacodynamics

No drug is free from toxic effect. Some of the examples of toxicities developed in response to administered drug in the human body are listed in the **Fig – Drug toxicities – few examples**.

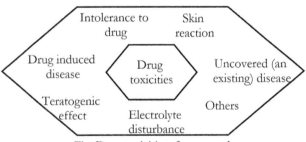

Fig: Drug toxicities -few example

16.6 Therapeutic index (TI)

It is essential to understand the therapeutic value of an administered drug by determining the margin of safety that exists between the dose needed for the desired effect and the dose that produces unwanted and possibly dangerous side effects.

Therapeutic index (also called therapeutic ratio) is the ratio between dosage of a drug that causes a lethal effect and the dosage that causes therapeutic effect. This pharmacodynamic parameter helps in estimating the safety profile of a drug i.e., how safe or toxic a drug is.

Lethal dose (LD) = dose of a drug which produces the lethal (killing) effect

Effective dose (ED) = dose of a drug which produces the desired/therapeutic effect

Thus, the median lethal dose and the median effective dose are arrived at as explained below:

Median lethal dose (LD_{50}) = dose which produces lethal (killing) effect in the half (50%) of a population tested

Median effective dose (ED50) = dose which produces the desired/therapeutic effect in half (50%) of a population tested

$$\text{Therapeutic Index} = \frac{\text{Median Lethal Dose (LD50)}}{\text{Median Effective Dose (ED50)}}$$

LD50 could also be replaced with Toxic dose (TD50).

Toxic dose (TD50) = dose which produces toxic effect in half (50%) of a population tested

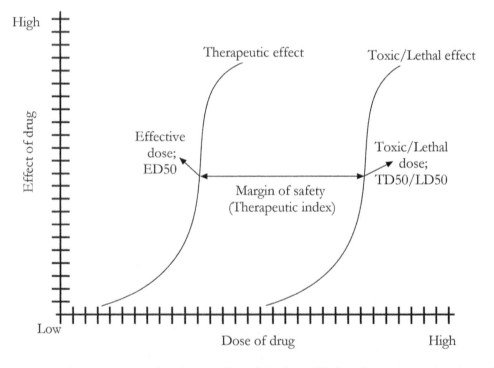

Therapeutic index presents an idea about safety of the drug. Higher the therapeutic index, safer is the drug.

16.7 Therapeutic Window

Therapeutic window is a range of doses that produces therapeutic effect without causing any significant harm in patients. It can be quantified by therapeutic index.

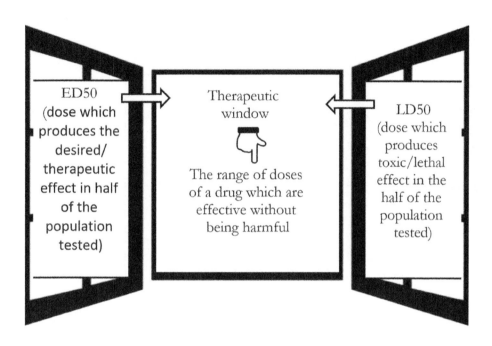

Generally, the therapeutic window is a ratio between minimum effective concentration (MEC) to the minimum toxic concentration (MTC). The levels of drug should always be in between minimum effective concentration (MEC) and minimum toxic concentration (MTC) in order to provide risk free therapeutic effects. If any drug crosses MTC then it will definitely produce toxic effects and if a drug is unable to beat the MEC then it will fail to produce therapeutic effect.

16.8 Pharmacokinetics

Pharmacokinetics is the study of movement of an administered drug into, through, and out of the body. It measures the time taken by drug to change in its concentration through different processes such as absorption (A), distribution (D), metabolism (M) and excretion (E) in a living system [refer to the **Fig – Pharmacokinetics**].

16.9 Absorption (of drug)

Absorption of administered drug into the body system is required for showing the effect of the drug. It is the movement of administered drug from the site of administration to the systematic circulation.

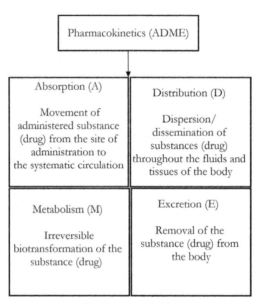

Fig: Pharmacokinetics

16.10 Factors influencing the rate of absorption

Factors which can impact the rate of absorption of administered drug in the living body are mentioned in **Fig – Factors determining rate of absorption**.

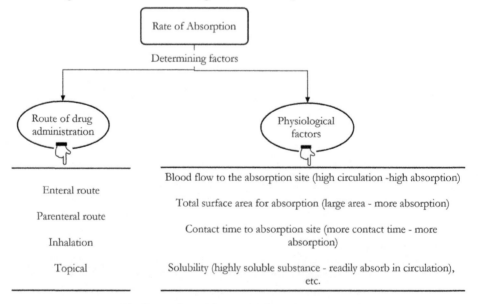

Fig: Factors determining rate of absorption

16.11 Route of drug administration

A drug will produce its effect only when it enters the body. The path taken by the drug to get into the body is known as the route of drug administration. Route of drug administration can be classified as depicted in the **Fig – Types of Routes of drug administration.**

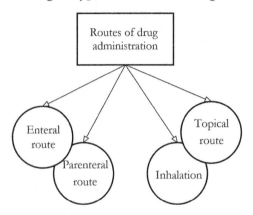

Fig: Types of routes of drug administration

Different types of routes of administration have been explained below:

16.12 Enteral route

It refers to anything involving alimentary tract (from mouth to the rectum). Different types of enteral routes are described in the **Fig – Types of Enteral route.**

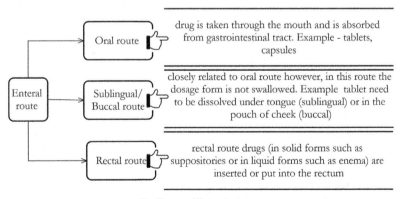

Fig: Types of Enteral route

(Suppositories are prepared by mixing medicine with a wax-like substance to form a semi-solid, bullet shaped form that will melt after insertion into the rectum.)

16.13 First-pass effect

It is a process in which a drug administered by mouth, and it is absorbed from the gastrointestinal tract and transported via the portal vein to the liver, where it is metabolized. As a result, in some cases only a small proportion of the active drug reaches the systemic circulation and its intended target tissue. It is also known as first-pass metabolism or presystemic metabolism. First-pass metabolism can be bypassed by giving the drug via sublingual or buccal routes.

16.14 Parenteral route

It refers to any route of administration outside of or beside the alimentary tract. This route of administration usually shows their effects more quickly. This route includes "Injections" (refer to the **Fig – Types of Injections**) which takes the drug directly into the tissue fluid or blood.

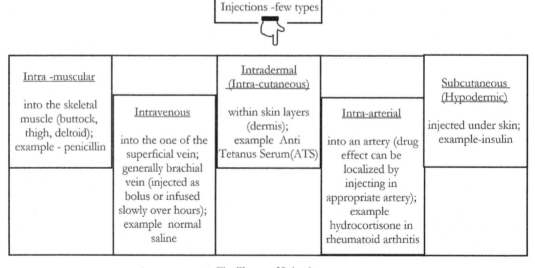

Intra-muscular		Intradermal (Intra-cutaneous)		Subcutaneous (Hypodermic)
into the skeletal muscle (buttock, thigh, deltoid); example - penicillin	Intravenous	within skin layers (dermis); example Anti Tetanus Serum(ATS)	Intra-arterial	injected under skin; example-insulin
	into the one of the superficial vein; generally brachial vein (injected as bolus or infused slowly over hours); example normal saline		into an artery (drug effect can be localized by injecting in appropriate artery); example hydrocortisone in rheumatoid arthritis	

Fig: Types of Injections

16.15 Inhalation

It refers to administration of the drug through the respiratory system in the form of gas, vapor or powder (refer to the **Fig – Types of Inhalation**). Through this route, the drug can pass directly into the lungs. Drugs forms used in this method include volatile drugs and gases. Example – aerosols like salbutamol

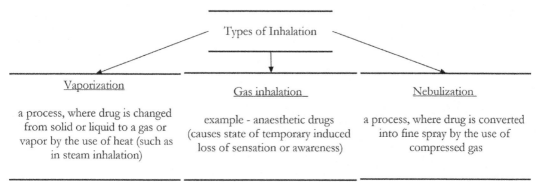

Fig: Types of Inhalation

16.16 Topical route

It refers to the application of drug to the external surfaces, the skin and the mucous membranes. Effects of topical route can be local or systematic (refer to the **Fig – Effects of Topical route** and **Fig – Different types of Topical routes**).

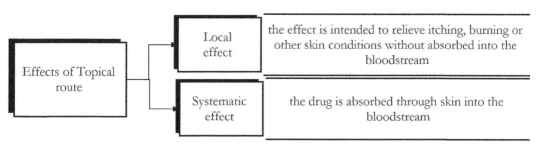

Fig: Effects of Topical route

16.17 Distribution (of drug)

Post absorption in the body, the drug will be distributed throughout the body. Distribution is the process by which a drug reversibly leaves the blood stream and enters the body's extracellular fluid and/or the cells or tissues.

The drugs are present in free or bound form inside the body (note: only the free drug is able to exert its effect). The administered drug is carried by the blood to the target site for drug action and to other tissues as well, where drug may produce side effects/adverse reactions. The rate and extent of distribution of an administered drug varies from site to site inside the body.

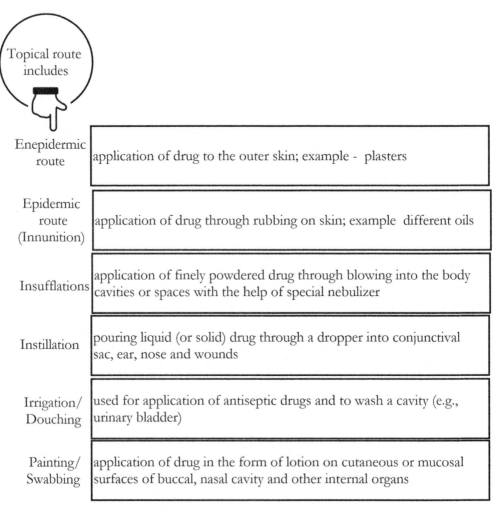

Fig: Different types of Topical routes

16.18 Factors influencing the rate of drug distribution

Drug distribution depends on the physicochemical properties of the administered drug and on the characteristics of body system of a patient who is receiving the drug. Hence, distribution of absorbed drug into body can be impacted by various factors and these influencing factors can be related to the body or to the administered drug (refer to the **Fig – Factors affecting distribution of administered drug inside human body**).

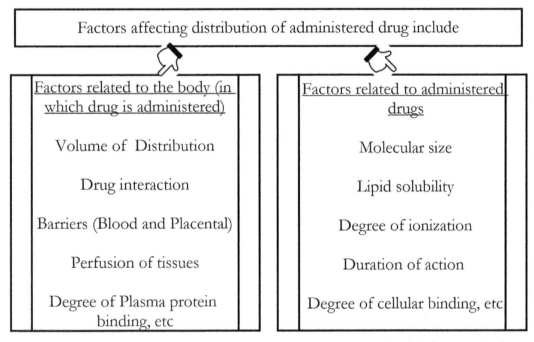

Fig: Factors affecting distribution of administered drug inside human body

Factors related to body	
Volume of Distribution	describes details about distribution of drug in the body
Drug Interaction	occurs when more than one drug administered simultaneously or administered drug interacts with endogenous substance
Barriers	Blood brain barrier and Placental barrier allow passage of selective substances
Perfusion of tissues	Well perfused tissues such as brain, heart allows rapid uptake of drug and hence drug gets distributed to these areas first while poorly perfused tissue such as adipose tissue, muscle tissue allow slow uptake of the drug and hence, drug arrives to these tissues later.
Plasma protein binding	administered drug can have affinity for proteins present in plasma (blood); e.g., acidic drug binds to plasma albumin

Factors related to drug	
Molecular size	smaller the size, more is the distribution and vice versa
Lipid solubility	greater the lipid solubility, higher the affinity for fat tissues; e.g., drugs can be held in adipose tissue
Degree of ionization	drugs are weak acid/base when they are getting distributed in the system; ionized drug can be confined in certain location inside body
Duration of action	Can be prolonged by presence of bound form of drug; when free drug is released from the body, bound drug can become free (from protein binding) to show action
Cellular binding	different drugs have different affinity for different cells

16.19 Volume of distribution (V_D)

Any administered drug, inside a living body, acts as a solute and the tissues of that living body act as solvents for that solute. Different tissues possess different specificities which will cause different concentrations of the drug within each group. Therefore, the chemical characteristics of a drug will determine its distribution within a body. For example, a liposoluble drug will tend to accumulate in body fat and water-soluble drugs will tend to accumulate in extracellular fluids.

The volume of distribution (V_D)determines the degree of distribution of a drug into various body compartments and tissues. It can be defined as the hypothetical volume of body fluid that would be required to dissolve the amount of drug, needed to achieve the same concentration in the blood.

In other words, the volume of distribution is the theoretical volume that a drug would have to occupy (if it were uniformly distributed), to provide the same concentration as it currently is in blood plasma.

Volume of distribution can be determined from the following formula:

$$(V_D) = (Ab)/(Cp)$$

Where:

(Ab) is total amount of the drug in the body and

(Cp) is the drug's plasma concentration

As the value of (Ab) is equivalent to the dose of the drug that has been administered, the formula shows us that there is an inversely proportional relationship between (V_D) and (Cp). That is, that the greater (Cp), is the lower (V_D) will be and vice versa.

Thus, the volume of distribution relates to the amount of a drug in the blood to the concentration measured in a body fluid. It provides the information on distribution of the drug in the body. A higher V_D indicates a greater amount of tissue distribution.

16.20 Metabolism (of drug)

Biotransformation of drugs to more hydrophilic molecules is required process for the elimination of the administered drug substance from the body. Drug alteration in a living system is known as "biotransformation" where body changes the chemical structure of a drug to another form called a "metabolite". The main objective of metabolism (biotransformation) of a drug is to facilitate the excretion of the drug from the body i.e., conversion of lipophilic drugs into hydrophilic compounds (conversion of non-excretable into excretable forms). Drug biotransformation, generally into more polar compounds, readily excreted from the body through urine or faeces.

16.21 Methods of Biotransformation (Metabolism)

Drug inside the body can be metabolized through synthetic and non-synthetic reactions (refer to the **Fig – Methods of Biotransformation**). Through metabolism, administered drug will either become more active or completely inactive. Major part of drug metabolism takes place in the liver as enzymes which supports the metabolic reactions are concentrated in liver.

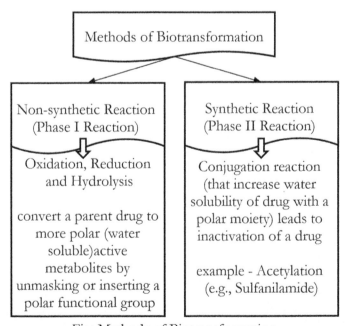

Fig: Methods of Biotransformation

Metabolites produced in synthetic reactions are more polar and thus more readily excreted by the kidneys (in urine) and the liver (in bile) than those formed in non-synthetic reactions. There are possibilities that few drugs undergo only phase I or phase II reactions. Hence, the classification of metabolic reactions reflects functional rather than sequential.

Rate of drug metabolism vary from person to person. Some individuals metabolize a drug so rapidly that therapeutically effective blood and tissue concentrations are not achieved. On the other hand, some individuals metabolize a drug so slow that usual doses have toxic effects. Factors affecting metabolism includes genetic factors, coexisting disorders, drug interactions, etc.

16.22 Excretion (of drug)

The process of removal of metabolic wastes from the living body is called excretion. Excretion is the passage out of systematically absorbed drug. Drugs may be excreted in an active or inactive form.

16.23 Types of Excretion

Kidney is considered the main excretory organ which does excretion through different processes (refer to the **Fig – Types of excretion**). Other routes for excretion include Lungs, Skin, Liver or Glandular structure such as salivary gland, lacrimal gland, etc. (Note: Renal refers to kidneys)

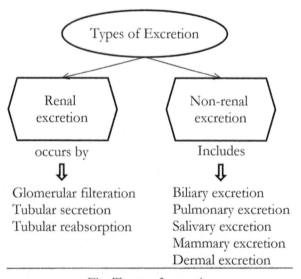

Fig: Types of excretion

Some drugs can be excreted without metabolism i.e., in unchanged form (original dosage form), whereas some drugs undergo metabolism process and excreted as metabolites. The kidneys excrete majority of water-soluble substances. The biliary system helps in excretion of drugs that are not reabsorbed from the gastrointestinal tract. Intestine, saliva, sweat, breast milk and lungs contribution are very less such as excretion of small concentration of drug through breast milk of lactating women (which may affect breastfeeding infant), volatile anesthetic drugs can be exhaled via the lungs, etc.

16.24 Fate of drug in the body

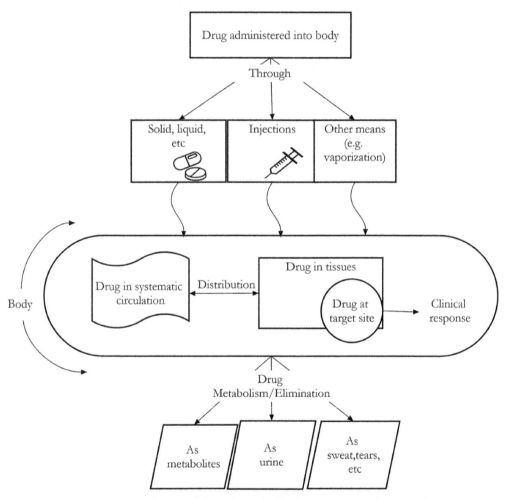

Fig: Fate of an administered drug inside the body-summerized overview

16.25 Drug – short introduction

Drug is a chemical substance used in the treatment, cure, prevention or diagnosis or used to otherwise enhance physical or mental well-being. In a diseased condition, the equilibrium of body gets disturbed which can be restored by the administration of correct drug.

16.26 Drug Nomenclature

A drug can have several names. Drug nomenclature is the systematic naming of drugs (especially pharmaceutical drugs). Generally, the drug names can be classified into three categories (refer to the **Fig – Drug Nomenclature**).

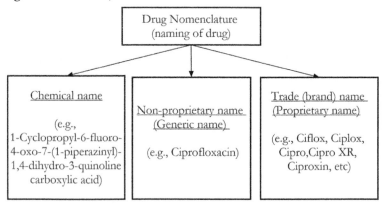

Fig: Drug Nomenclature

16.27 Chemical name

Important points related to chemical name is mentioned in the **Fig – Chemical name**.

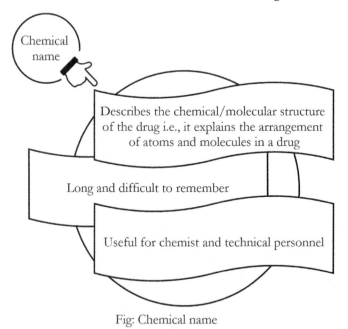

Fig: Chemical name

16.28 Non-proprietary name (Generic name)

Important points related to Non-proprietary name (Generic name) is listed in the **Fig – Non-proprietary name (Generic name).**

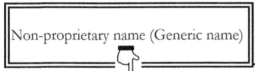

Non-proprietary name (Generic name)

Short and meaningful name of the drug

Not subject to proprietary rights

An international non-proprietary name(INN) is an official generic and non-proprietary name given to a pharmaceutical drug or active ingredient.

International non-proprietary names enable communication more precise and accurate by providing a unique standard name for each active ingredient. It helps in avoiding prescribing errors.

World Health Organization(WHO) approves the INN.

A generic drug name is not capitalized. Example - atorvastatin

A generic drug is a pharmaceutical drug that is equivalent to a brand-name product in dosage, strength, route of administration, quality, performance and intended use.

This can be done when patent (reserved by the original manufacturer) for a particular drug is expired.

Fig: Non-proprietary name (Generic name)

16.29 Trade (brand) name (Proprietary name)

Important points related to Trade (brand) name (Proprietary name) are listed in the **Fig – Trade (brand) name (Proprietary name).**

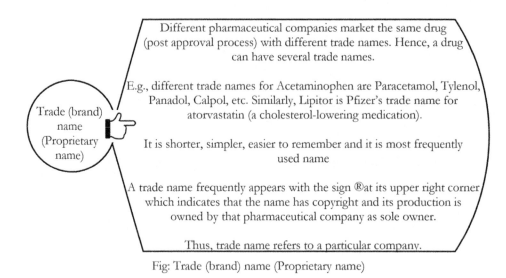

Fig: Trade (brand) name (Proprietary name)

16.30 Drug Nomenclature - Examples

Chemical Name	Non-proprietary name	Trade name
N-acetyl-p-aminophenol	paracetamol acetaminophen	Tylenol
(RS)-2-(4-(2-methylpropyl)phenyl)propanoic acid	ibuprofen	Motrin
(2R,3S,4R,5R,8R,10R,11R,12S,13S,14R) -13-[(2,6-dideoxy-3-C-methyl-3-O-methyl-α-L-ribo-hexopyranosyl)oxy]-2-ethyl-3,4,10-trihydroxy-3,5,6,8,10,12,14-heptamethyl-11-[[3,4,6-trideoxy-3-(dimethylamino)-β-D-xylo-hexopyranosyl] oxy]-1-oxa-6-azacyclopentadecan-15-one	azithromycin	Zithromax
2-acetoxybenzoic acid	acetylsalicylic acid	Aspirin
2-(diphenylmethoxy)-N,N-dimethylethylamine hydrochloride	diphenhydramine	Benadryl
(3R,5R)-7-[2-(4-fluorophenyl)-3-phenyl-4-(phenylcarbamoyl)-5-propan-2-ylpyrrol-1-yl]-3,5-dihydroxyheptanoic acid	atorvastatin	Lipitor

Suggestion: Remember at least few names of medicines related to common diseases. It may be helpful for interview purpose and for studying clinical research as well.

Example –

Antihistamine (suppress histamine induced allergic reactions) – Cetirizine

Anti – anxiety drug (used for the treatment of symptoms of anxiety) – Diazepam, Alprazolam

Chapter 17

SHORT NOTES

17.1 Introduction

These short notes are crisp content about few important topics which can augment the reader's knowledge further in the field of clinical research.

17.2 Key responsibilities of key players in Clinical Trial (Clinical Research)

There are a number of responsibilities associated with each player of a clinical trial. Some important responsibilities associated with some important players are listed below:

17.3 Key responsibilities of Regulatory authority (agency)

- Overall responsible to promote, ensure and monitor compliance by approved ethics committees in a country with relevant legislation, regulations and guidelines

- Responsible to review clinical trials of both non-registered medicinal substances and new indications of registered medicinal substances

- Possesses the authority to close down an ongoing trial in the case there are serious breaches of Good Clinical Practice

- Ensures that the drugs available in the country fulfils the necessary requirements for safety, quality and efficacy

- Ensures the presence of a regulatory system which confirms that all clinical trials which is needed to be conducted in the country must have registered with competent authority

- Reviews all the documents (containing clinical and non-clinical data) before approving the marketing of a new drug in any country to ensure the efficacy and safety of the drug in human

17.4 Key responsibilities of Sponsor

- Investigator(s) selection and introducing him/her to the necessary information which are required to conduct the clinical trial

- To ensure all needed approvals and ethic review(s) are taken for the trial

- To prepare and submit the clinical trial application(s) and amendment(s) to the appropriate regulatory authorities

- To ensure all significant new information in a trial is reported promptly and in timely manner to ethics committee and regulatory authority

- To ensure proper monitoring of the clinical study and also to check the study is in accordance with GCP and applicable regulations

- To ensure compliance with labelling, reporting and record-keeping requirements

- To abstain from engaging in promotional activities and other prohibited activities such as commercializing an investigational medical device, etc.

17.5 Key responsibilities of Principal Investigator (PI)

- Primary responsibility to ensure the ethical conduct of the research trial/study

- To protect the rights, safety and welfare of subjects in a clinical trial/study

- To ensure that informed consent is properly obtained from clinical trial subjects

- To work as team leader for clinical research team (in case there is team for conducting a trial) and to ensure that the trial is conducted according to the protocol

- To ensure integrity and quality of the clinical data

- To ensure proper record-keeping and reporting requirements are met, etc.

17.6 Key responsibilities of Sub-Investigator / Co-Investigator

- May perform all or some of the PI functions, but they are not primarily responsible for the clinical trial/study

- To work under the supervision of the PI

- To handle study–related procedures and to take part in making important study-related decisions in compliance with the ethical conduct of the study, etc.

17.7 Key responsibilities of Human subjects (Study Participants)

- To cooperate properly and fully with study procedures

- To follow all clinical study directions provided by research investigator/staff

- To take prescribed medications as per instructions

- To inform all happenings which may be relevant to study

- To answer to the questions (asked by investigator/other research staff) truthfully

- To be clear with all doubts related to study by asking questions to the research staffs, etc.

17.8 Key responsibilities of IRB/IEC

- To review all study-related materials before and during the trial

- To ensure that trial is taking place in accordance with national and/or local regulations, as well as with ICH good clinical practices (GCPs) guidelines

- To safeguard the rights, safety, and well-being of all trial subjects (Special attention should be paid to trials that may include vulnerable subjects)

- To review the appropriateness of the clinical trial protocol

- To review the risks and benefits to study participants

- To ensure that clinical trial participants are exposed to minimal risks in relation to any benefits that might result from the research, etc.

17.9 Key responsibilities of Clinical Research Coordinator (CRC)

- To coordinate the daily activities of clinical trial/study

- To work closely with investigator and research team to ensure that all protocol required procedures and visits occur according to protocol specified guidelines

- To be involved in managing participant enrolment and ensuring compliance with the protocol and other applicable regulations

- To create source document

- To help in the assessment of toxicities/adverse events and reporting of serious adverse events as per IRB and sponsor requirements, etc.

17.10 Key responsibilities of Clinical Research Associate (CRA)

- To assess clinical trial/study site for its potential
- To get involved in the implementation of clinical trial related processes
- To ensure that the study staff get proper training to conduct the trial related activities properly
- To monitor the trial throughout the specified duration
- To get involved in writing visit reports, filing and collecting trial documentation and reports
- To look into the compliance related matters
- To ensure the trial is running smoothly through maintaining the consistency with sponsor's content
- To ensure quality of the data produced during research
- To get involved in closing process of the study, etc.

  {CRA is also known as "Monitor"}

  Other players involved in trial can be biostatistician, data mangers, etc.

17.11 Essential Documents

Essential Documents are those documents that individually and collectively permit evaluation of the conduct of a trial and the quality of the data produced. Essential Documents also serve a number of other important purposes. Few are listed below:

- Demonstrate the compliance of the investigator, sponsor, and monitor with all applicable regulatory requirements and GCP
- Assist in the successful management of the study by the investigator, sponsor, and monitor
- Confirm the validity of the conduct of the clinical investigation and the integrity of the data collected.

The ICH E6 consolidation guide for GCP, categorizes these documents into three parts, depending upon the stage of the study during which they would normally be generated:

- Prior to commencement of clinical trial; example – IB, Signed Protocol
- During the conduct of the trial; example – updates – IB, ICF

- After completion (or termination) of the trial; example – audit certificate, final closeout report

It is acceptable to combine some of the documents, as long as the individual elements are readily identifiable.

Filing essential documents at the investigator/institution and sponsor sites in a timely manner can greatly assist in the successful management of a trial. During audit by audit team appointed by sponsor and inspection by regulatory authority, essential documents can also be audited to confirm the validity of trial conduct and the integrity and quality of data produced.

17.12 Good manufacturing practice (GMP)

Good manufacturing practice (GMP) is a system for ensuring that medicinal products are consistently produced and controlled according to quality standards. GMP was promulgated by the US Food and Drug Administration under the authority of the Federal Food, Drug, and Cosmetic Act. It is designed to minimize the risks involved in any pharmaceutical production that cannot be eliminated through testing the final product. The main risks are:

- Unexpected contamination of products

- Causing damage to health or even death

- Incorrect labels on containers, which could mean that patients receive the wrong medicine; insufficient or too much active ingredient, resulting in ineffective treatment or adverse effects.

Good manufacturing practice guidelines provide guidance for manufacturing, testing, and quality assurance in order to ensure that a food or drug product is safe for human consumption. It covers all aspects of production; from the starting materials, premises and equipment to the training and personal hygiene of staff. Detailed, written procedures are essential for each process in order to ensure the production of quality product.

GMP ensures the production of high quality medicinal products. The manufacturing companies must comply with GMP regulations otherwise their manufacturing authorisation may get cancelled.

GMP is also sometimes referred to as "cGMP". The "c" stands for "current," which represents that manufacturers must use current technologies and systems in order to comply with the regulation. The approval process for new drug and generic drug marketing applications includes a review of the manufacturer's compliance with the cGMP.

17.13 Good Laboratory Practice (GLP)

Good Laboratory Practice is defined as "a quality system concerned with the organisational process and the conditions under which non-clinical health and environmental safety studies are planned, performed, monitored, recorded, archived and reported."

The purpose of the Principles of Good Laboratory Practice is to promote the development of quality test data and provide a tool to ensure a sound approach to the management of laboratory studies, including conduct, reporting and archiving.

GLP was first introduced in New Zealand and Denmark in 1972, and later in the US in 1978 in response to the Industrial BioTest Labs scandal. It was followed a few years later by the Organization for Economic Co-operation and Development (OECD) Principles of GLP in 1992. The OECD has since helped promulgate GLP to many countries.

Important features of GLP

- GLP only applies to non-clinical studies and it sets out the requirements for the appropriate management of nonclinical safety studies.

- GLP does not apply to the clinical studies.

- GLP is a quality management system which defines a set of quality standards for study conduct, data collection, and reporting of results.

- GLP is not a scientific management system i.e. it does not directly concern with the scientific design of the studies.

The scientific design may be based on test guidelines and its scientific value is judged by the (Drug) Regulatory Authority that provides marketing authorisation. However, adherence to GLP will remove many sources of error and uncertainty, adding to the overall credibility of the study.

GLP Principles help to define and standardise the planning, performance, recording, reporting, monitoring and archiving processes within research institutions. Since all these aspects are of equal importance for compliance with GLP Principles, it is not permissible to partially implement GLP requirements and still claim GLP compliance.

The study director plays a critical role in preclinical drug or medical device testing. He/she is responsible for overseeing the study from beginning to end to ensure that all Good Laboratory Practices (GLP) are met and that the outcome of the study is valid and reliable. He/she will assert this at the end of the study in his/her dated and signed GLP Compliance Statement which is included in the study report.

17.14 Data monitoring committee (DMC) or Data Safety Monitoring Board (DSMB)

A data monitoring committee (DMC) or data safety monitoring board (DSMB) is an independent group of experts who monitor patient safety and treatment efficacy data while a clinical trial is ongoing. They review the accumulated data from one or more ongoing clinical trials on a regular basis and advise the sponsor about:

- The continued safety of the trial participants

- The continued validity of the trial

- The continued scientific merit of the trial

FDA does not require a DSMB for every study. That means, safety monitoring is must for all the clinical trials but it is not compulsory for all the trials to have an external body to monitor the safety concerns. For instance, "low risk" interventions, (e.g., physiotherapy trials), only internal monitoring can be sufficient. DSMBs are mainly required in studies where interim data analysis is important to ensure the safety of the study subjects.

Purpose of a DSMB:

- To ensure the safety of the study subjects

- To ensure the credibility of the trial and the validity of trial results

- To identify unacceptably slow rates of accrual

- To identify high rates of ineligibility determined after randomization

- To identify protocol violations that suggest clarification of changes to protocol are needed

- To identify unexpectedly high dropout rates that threaten the trial's ability to produce credible results

17.15 ClinicalTrials.gov

ClinicalTrials.gov is a registry and results database of publicly and privately supported clinical studies of human participants conducted around the world. Most of the records on ClinicalTrials.gov describe clinical trials.

ClinicalTrials.gov is a web-based resource maintained by National Library of Medicine (NLM) at the National Institutes of Health (NIH). This site furnishes patients, their family members, health care professionals, researchers, and the public with easy access to information on publicly and privately supported clinical studies on a wide range of diseases and conditions.

Typically, the sponsor or principal investigator of the clinical study provides and updates the details related to studies. Generally, at the start of the study, they submit the relevant details to the web site which gets updated throughout the study. In some cases, results of the study are submitted after the study ends. This Web site and database of clinical studies is commonly referred to as a "registry and results database."

17.16 Medical Device

According to FDA, a medical device is "an instrument, apparatus, implement, machine, contrivance, implant, in vitro reagent, or other similar or related article, including a component part, or accessory which is:

- recognized in the official National Formulary, or the United States Pharmacopoeia, or any supplement to them,

- intended for use in the diagnosis of disease or other conditions, or in the cure, mitigation, treatment, or prevention of disease, in man or other animals, or

- intended to affect the structure or any function of the body of man or other animals, and which does not achieve any of its primary intended purposes through chemical action within or on the body of man or other animals and which is not dependent upon being metabolized for the achievement of any of its primary intended purposes."

In simple words,

Any health care product that is intended for the diagnosis, prevention, or treatment of disease and does not primarily work by effecting a chemical change in the body.

Example - Diagnostic test kits, pacemakers, catheters, intraocular lens

Device Classification

Devices are classified into three categories:

- Class I devices - low risk that require general controls to assure safety and effectiveness

- Class II devices - moderate risk and are subject to both general and special controls

- Class III devices - high risk and are subject to the highest level of regulatory requirements

The FDA has exempted almost all Class I devices with the exception of some listed as "Reserved Devices" from the PMA requirements. Some Class II devices are now exempt from Pre-market notification requirements due to the 1997 FDA Modernization Act. All Class III devices and those that do not meet the criteria for exemption or a 510(k) require a PMA.

Medical devices distributed in the United States must comply with the following regulatory requirements:

- Establishment Registration

- Medical Device Listing

- Premarket Notification 510(k), unless exempt, or Premarket Approval (PMA)

- Investigational Device Exemption (IDE) for studies

- Quality Systems Regulation

- Labeling Requirements

- Medical Device Reporting (MDR)

Device development regulations are comprised of exceptions, exemptions, and special classifications. For example, devices being tested to determine consumer preference can be exempt if they are not intended to establish safety or effectiveness.

If a device manufacturer does not have a device that is exempt from the regulatory requirements they either have to complete a Pre-Market Notification 510(k) or a Premarket Approval (PMA). If the 510(k) or PMA requires clinical data to support the application, an Investigational Device Exemption (IDE) may also need to be filed.

17.17 Correlation study

- Correlation study aims to predict.

- Important features of correlation study are described below:

    I. It studies the relationship between two variables or investigates the degree of association between two variables. It determines whether two variables are correlated or not i.e. whether an increase or decrease in one variable corresponds to an increase or decrease in the other variable.

    II. It doesn't suggest causation however, it ponders the quality of connection between two variables and gives a sign of how one variable may foresee another.

III. Three sorts of Correlation are:

    ✓ <u>Positive correlation</u> – Both variables increase or decrease at the same time, e.g., More workout/exercise – more fat burn, lesser workout/exercise – lesser fat burn

    ✓ <u>Negative correlation</u> – The measure of one variable increases and the measure of other variable decreases, e.g., increase in smoking – deterioration in health

    ✓ <u>No correlation</u> –Indicates no correlation between two variables, e.g. screen size of the phone – no change in internet bill

- Correlation coefficient – it is numerical portrayal of the quality and direction of the relationship. It varies between +1 and -1. A value close to +1 indicates a strong positive correlation while a value close to -1 indicates strong negative correlation. A value near zero shows that the variables are not correlated.

- Results of correlation study can be plotted in graph.

17.18 In vitro studies, In vivo studies, Ex vivo studies, In silico studies

In vitro ("within the glass") studies

These tests conducted in a controlled environment (in the lab) outside of a living organism, usually in test tubes. Many experiments in cellular biology are conducted outside of organisms/cells.

One important disadvantage of in vitro experiments is that, results obtained from these experiments may not anticipate the complete and accurate effects on a whole organism i.e. these experiments fail to replicate the precise cellular conditions of an organism, particularly a microbe. Example - work on some cell line, which originally developed from the primary culture long time ago, is usually described as in vitro experiment.

In vivo ("within the living") studies

These experiments are conducted in a whole, living organism. In vivo testing is often employed over in vitro because it is better suited for observing the overall effects of an experiment on a living organism. Animal studies and clinical trials are examples of in vivo research.

Ex vivo ("out of the living") studies

These experiments are conducted in or on tissue from an organism in an external environment with minimal alteration of natural conditions. Ex vivo conditions allow experimentation on an organism's cells or tissues under more controlled conditions than is possible in in vivo experiments (in the intact organism), at the cost of altering the "natural" environment.

Example - ex vivo gene therapy means that cells are taken directly from the body, transduced with the gene in vitro and then returned to the body.

In silico studies ("in silicon") studies

This is an expression used to mean "performed on computer or via computer simulation."

It has begun to be used widely in studies, which predict how drugs interact with the body and with pathogens. For example, a 2009 study used software emulations to predict how certain drugs already on the market could treat multiple-drug-resistant and extensively drug-resistant strains of tuberculosis.

17.19 Patient Diary

A patient diary is a tool used during a clinical trial or in a disease treatment to assess the patient's condition (e.g. symptom severity, quality of life) or to measure treatment compliance. An electronic patient diary registers the data in a storage device and allows for automatically monitoring the time of data entry.

A patient diary is very helpful for patients in taking care of their own health by identifying the problem before they become worst and by taking required actions for the same.

Importance of Patient health diary:

- It primarily focuses on chronic disease conditions, such as diabetes, asthma, etc.
- It keeps track of physiological signs such as blood glucose, blood pressure, weight, etc.
- It reminds the importance of self-monitoring.
- It is used to help patients and healthcare professionals to assess symptoms and follow specific lifestyle changes.
- It may also take care of medications, in case patient needs to take many medicines in different times with some specifications (e.g., some with food and others not).
- Example - Diet diary, Sleep diary, Exercise diary, etc.
- Let's take the example of Food diary. This kind of diary keeps reminding the patient of:
  ✓ When to eat – time to eat; e.g., timings of small meals
  ✓ What to eat – food name; e.g., white rice or brown rice in lunch

✓ How to eat - cooking procedure; e.g., boiled food

✓ How much to eat – food quantity; e.g., two chapattis without oil in dinner, etc.

FDA guidance listed three reasons to collect the data reported by the patient (subject in case of an experiment):

• Some treatment effects are known only to the patient

• There is a desire to know the patient perspective about the effectiveness of a treatment

• Systematic assessment of the patient's perspective may provide valuable information that can be lost when that perspective is filtered through a clinician's evaluation of the patient's response to clinical interview questions

17.20 Evidence-based medicine (EBM)

Evidence-based medicine (EBM) is an approach to medical practice intended to optimize decision-making by emphasizing the use of evidence from well-designed and well-conducted research.

Evidence-based medicine consists of three key elements. They are:

• Research-based evidence

• Clinical expertise (i.e., the clinician's accumulated experience, knowledge, and clinical skills)

• Patient's values and preferences

In EBM, researchers chose the best sources for analysis through utilization of systematic reviews and meta-analyses. Thus, EBM helps researchers in discovering the best available evidence.

Important features of EBM:

• EBM integrates clinical experience and patient values with the best available research information

• EBM aims to increase the use of high quality clinical research in clinical decision making

• EBM seeks better evidence than traditional medicine does

EBM is all about making use of the best available information to answer the questions in clinical practice. EBM enables the clinicians to discover and evaluate the information available related to a topic in order to estimate its reliability and then to decide if they can use these results to their patients. EBM can be summarized in following steps:

- Construction of an explicit clinical question from a patient's problem

- Exploration of the available literature for relevant information

- Evaluation of the evidence for its validity and effectiveness

- Implementation of useful findings in clinical practice

Practicing evidence-based medicine is becoming an inevitable component of today's healthcare environment because this approach is able to provide improved quality of care, improved patient's satisfaction, and reduced healthcare costs. Some of the other important benefits of EBM are listed below:

- Assists healthcare providers in being up to date with standardized evidence based protocols

- Applies near real-time information to make healthcare decisions

- Enhances clarity regarding prescribed guidelines, responsibilities towards decisions making for healthcare, and values associated with quality of care

- Enhanced results

- Reduction in healthcare cost as care improves

- Patient feels safe with best available treatment

17.21 Clinical Implementation Tools

There are a number of tools used to implement clinical evidence into routine practice but no single or combination of tool has proven sufficient or completely effective. Some of the available tools are discussed below:

1) Provider based implementation tools - Some of the provider based implementation tools are mentioned below:

   ✓ Continuing Medical Education (CME) - It helps healthcare providers to maintain competence and learn about new and developing areas of medical field. It consists of educating methods that can affect clinical knowledge, skills, attitudes, practice patterns and patient outcomes.

   ✓ Clinical Guidelines - These are systematically developed statements to assist healthcare professionals and patients in situations to take decisions about appropriate healthcare for specific clinical circumstances.

   ✓ Academic Detailing (educational outreach, educational detailing, or educational visiting) - It is a kind of designed visits by trained personnel to health care providers.

Trained personnel present the clinical practitioner attuned training and technical assistance so that they (clinical practitioner) can use best practices in order to improve the quality of care and patient's outcomes. Apart from face-to-face, web-based and other technologies can also be used for academic detailing.

✓ Physician Audit and Feedback - This kind of audit and feedback can be helpful for healthcare providers to understand their own clinical practices and thereby improving the same.

2) Patient based implementation tools - This kind of tool is related to educate patient regarding self-management skills. This tool can work efficiently by the combined effort of healthcare providers and patients. It includes:

✓ Identifying issues from the common point of view of the patient and healthcare team

✓ Aiming at issues, setting appropriate objectives and developing action plans together

✓ Continuing self-management training and support services for patients

✓ Active follow up to reinforce the implementation of the care plan

This tool can result in output with significant improvements and it can also help in reducing the cost of treatment. For instance, patients (at appointments) presenting the health maintenance reminder card to their physicians, can impact positively the rate of screening of particular disease.

3) Community based implementation tools - Before proceeding with this tool, it is important to understand clearly and completely the culture and other important aspects of the community. For the success of community based implementation tool, it is must to have good community partnership and relationships. Community Health Advisor (CHA) model is one the example of this tool.

✓ Community Health Advisor (CHA) model - It is a health improvement tool which has been implemented throughout the world to help public health leaders, decisionmakers, and others who are seeking to improve community health. It delivers tailored information about the potential health and cost impact of implementing evidence-based interventions.

4) Organization based implementation tools - Some organization based tools are as follows:

✓ System reengineering - The ultimate objective of healthcare systems is to demonstrate positive changes to patient outcomes and cost savings. In system reengineering, redesigning of the entire system may be taken in consideration instead of small changes to clinical microsystems.

✓ Computer based system - This kind of system may provide clinical decision support by assisting the healthcare providers with (a) making a diagnosis, (b) choosing among alternative treatments or (c) deciding upon a particular drug dosage.

✓ Pay for Performance (P4P) - A kind of financial rewards to the healthcare providers who achieve, improve or exceed their performance against certain benchmarks in health care services. It is also known as "value-based purchasing".

17.22 Product Monograph

A Product Monograph is a factual, scientific document on a drug product that, devoid of promotional material, describes the properties, claims, indications and conditions of use of the drug and contains any other information that may be required for optimal, safe and effective use of the drug.

The Product Monograph consists of three parts:

• Part 1 - Health Professional Information, that is (i.e.) prescribing information;

• Part 2 - Scientific Information; and

• Part 3 - Consumer Information.

Product monograph is an important part of the drug review process. Once authorized by health authority, product monograph is used by the drug manufacturer or sponsor to inform physicians, pharmacists, dentists, nurses and other health care professionals about the appropriate use of the drug. It also serves as a standard against which all promotional material distributed by the sponsor about the drug can be compared.

17.23 Pharmacogenomics

Pharmacogenomics - Pharmacology (the science of drugs) + Genomics (the study of genes and their functions)

Pharmacogenomics is the study of the role of the genome in drug response. It describes how genes affect a person's response to drugs. It helps in developing effective, safe medications and doses that will be tailored to a person's genetic makeup.

Once drug is administered to the body, body system processes the drug and body also gives some response to that drug. Different body systems (of different people) respond differently (good response, bad response, neutral response) to a single medicine due to their different genetic model. In the study of Pharmacogenomics, scientists study the genomic base to determine the influence of genetic factors on the given response by the body to the administered drug. With the help of these studies, scientists can produce customized and personalized drugs that can render more benefits and less side effects and risks to the individuals.

17.24 Pharmacoepidemiology

Pharmacoepidemiology is the study of the uses and effects of drugs in well-defined populations. It provides an estimate of the probability of beneficial effects of a drug in a population and the probability of adverse effects.

Pharmacoepidemiology is also helpful in studying and understanding drug safety issues. For example - confirmation and quantification of the relation between NSAID treatment and gastrointestinal ulceration and bleeding.

Pharmacoepidemiology is a bridge between clinical pharmacology and epidemiology. (Clinical pharmacology is the study of effect of drugs on clinical humans and Epidemiology is the study of the distribution and determinants of diseases and other health states in populations.)

Pharmacoepidemiology sometimes also involves the conduct and evaluation of programmatic efforts to improve medication use on a population basis. Pharmacoepidemiologic studies are largely based on observational rather than experimental data.

17.25 Me too medicine

'Me too' medicines are products which have more or less identical clinical outcomes to existing medicines. They are compounds structurally very similar to already known medicines that have an identical mechanism of action with only minor pharmacological differences. They can present some benefits, like providing more therapeutic options and in a few cases, lead to price reductions, but also involve disadvantages, like diminishing innovation in pioneering treatments.

First-in-class drug, Me-too drug & Generic drug

- First-in-class drug – In this type of drug, both the drug molecule and the target are novel. These products contain compound that acts on a specific and new target. These drugs use a new and unique mechanism of action for treating a medical condition. These products are often referred to as innovative drug.

- Me-too drug – In this type of drug, the molecule is novel but the target is not novel. These products contain compounds (usually from competing companies) that act on the same target where the first-in-class compound acts. Me-too drug is also known as "Follow-on drug".

- Generic drug- In this type of drug, neither the molecule nor the target is novel. These products contain the same active ingredient as a previously marketed product (innovative drug) contains.

The pharmaceutical companies compete with each other for development of medicinal product, and when one of them gets success in discovering a significant new drug, the others try to quickly produce their own versions of the new drug. Although they are based on the same breakthrough (hence the expression "me too"), the new versions are sufficiently different in some ways from the original one so that they can be patented in their own right.

Advantages of Me-too drug:

- Some me-too drugs are better than innovative drug; e.g., Simvastatin (me-too drug) is more effective than Lovastatin (innovative drug)

- Increased choice between drugs (me-too and innovative drug)

- May lead to significant price reduction for healthcare

Disadvantages of Me-too drug:

- May contain unacceptable benefit/risk ratio; e.g., Baycol (me-too drug) was withdrawn from the market due to excess number of cases of Rhabdomyolysis (a condition in which breakdown of muscle tissue occurs that releases a damaging protein into the blood)

- Reduces the motivation to invest in developing the innovative drug (me-too drug only needs additional costs of product development, testing, and promotion)

- May consume more resources than they (me-too drugs) are worth

Chapter 18

ACTIVITY ASSIGNMENTS

- What should an interested participant consider before participating in a trial?

- What kind of preparation is required to be done by a potential participant who is planning to meet with a researcher?

- Can a participant continue to take medication prescribed to him/her by a primary health care provider while in a trial?

- Find out the best skills which should be possessed by a researcher.

- Find out the difference between efficacy and effectiveness.

- Find out the reason behind taking healthy volunteers (generally) in the phase I of clinical trial.

- Find out the difference between verification and validation.

- Find out about surgical clinical trials.

- Do Placebos expire?

Chapter 19

CAREERS IN CLINICAL RESEARCH

19.1 Learnings from the chapter

- *Relevant competencies/skills required to make a progressive career in the field of Clinical Research*

- *Selection process followed by companies to recruit professionals for fresher jobs*

- *Personality traits which determine the overall employability chances of a candidate*

- *Various Job roles/positions and the respective role summary*

- *Subject related interview questions*

19.2 Introduction

Clinical Research is one of the most happening fields. To make a career in this industry, the aspirant must hold a Bachelor degree in Science domain (qualification in pharmacy, life science, bioscience, Biotechnology, Microbiology, medicine etc). There is a high demand for clinical research professionals in the industry. This chapter focuses on the relevant competencies with respect to the career aspect for the aspirants looking for career pathways in Clinical Research industry.

19.3 Career pathways in clinical research

A snapshot of career pathways for the aspirants of Clinical Research Field has been depicted in the **Fig – Clinical Research Career Pathways – Industry – Organization Types – Jobs**.

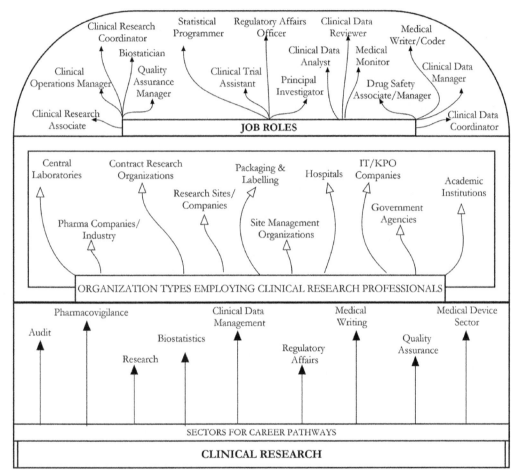

Fig: Clinical Research Career Pathways - Industry - Organization Types - Job

19.4 Different job roles in nutshell

The summary of job role for few of the job positions in Clinical Research domain have been depicted here:

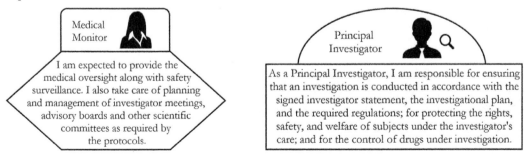

Clinical Research
Coordinator

I am responsible for
conducting clinical trials at
clinical trial sites in accordance
with the protocol, ICH-GCP
and other regulatory
requirements.

Clinical Trial
Assistant

As a Clinical Trial Assistant (CTA)
I am expected to assist the clinical
research teams in ensuring that the most
effective and efficient conduct of clinical research
by providing administration and project tracking
support.

Clinical Data
Reviewer

I am expected to work with data review assignments
during which, I do a point by point data check and
validation of data collected during clinical trials.
I support the data management team wherever
necessary and interface with them for any query
resolution.

Clinical Operations
Manager

As a clinical operations manager, I oversees the routine clinical
activities of a health-care institution (such as a medical facility,
a hospital or a research lab). I need to ensures that the facility
and its employees adhere to the required clinical protocols and
government regulations. I also need to monitor the work of
clinical operations personnel thereby ensuring that employees
conform to policies and regulatory guidelines.

Clinical Research
Associate

As a clinical research associate (CRA), I am resposible
for setting up, tracking and completing the clinical
trials. I collect the data and organize the data which is
compiled during studies and trials. I coordinate and
process the results gained from long-term testing of
drugs, products and medical procedures.

Clinical Data Manager

I am accountable for collection of data from various
medical research projects (for example clinical and
pharmaceutical trials). I am also expected to create
the database systems that meet the needs of research
team for the data storage/analysis.

Clinical Data
Coordinator

I am expected to handle the clinical info
such as patient records, appointments,
studies, and other official documents. I
also coordinate activities with respect to
administrative tasks concerning
recording of data for study and
validation.

Drug Safety
Associate/Officer

As a drug safety associate/officer, I take care of the
review, evaluation and management of adverse event
reports arising out of clinical trials (in accordance with
the specified guidelines and other applicable regulations).
I also support the medical review team whenever
necessary.

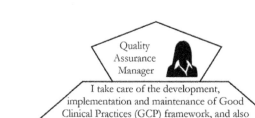

Quality Assurance Manager

I take care of the development, implementation and maintenance of Good Clinical Practices (GCP) framework, and also work towards ensuring the execution of established requirements/standards

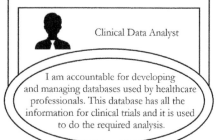

Clinical Data Analyst

I am accountable for developing and managing databases used by healthcare professionals. This database has all the information for clinical trials and it is used to do the required analysis.

Statistical Programmer

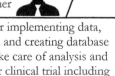

I am responsibile for implementing data, performing validation and creating database information. I also take care of analysis and reporting activities for clinical trial including the planning, supervision, implementation and maintenance of clinical programming processes

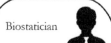

Biostatician

I am expected to contribute in all areas of a clinical research study starting with experimental design, sample size considerations, biostatistic methodology etc resulting in proper and meaningful data analysis, interpretation and meaningful comprehensive conclusion thereby helping towards research study reports/manuscript preparation and scientific publication.

Medical Writer

I work with medical and technical professionals to develop documents for government review. I am expected to have a very good understanding of medical terminology as I use scientific knowledge and writing skills to effectively communicate as required. I do scientific medical writing (related to medical studies). I also do writing with respect to drug trials and regulatory documents. I can also work for marketing medical writing, which includes news releases and advertising copy for a wider audience.

Regulatory Affairs Executive/Officer

As a Regulatory affairs officer, I act as a bridge between the company and regulatory authorities. Thus, I need to ensure that products are manufactured and distributed in compliance with appropriate regulations. I also ensure that products such as cosmetics, pharmaceuticals, and veterinary medicines meet legislative requirements.

19.5 General Competencies for clinical research aspirants/professionals

Competence is the ability of an individual to do a job properly. A competency is a set of defined behaviours that provide a structured guide enabling the identification, evaluation and development of the behaviours in individual employees. Competencies are the measurable or observable knowledge, skills, abilities, and behaviours (KSABs) critical to successful job performance.

Listed below are some important competency areas which the aspirants need to focus on.

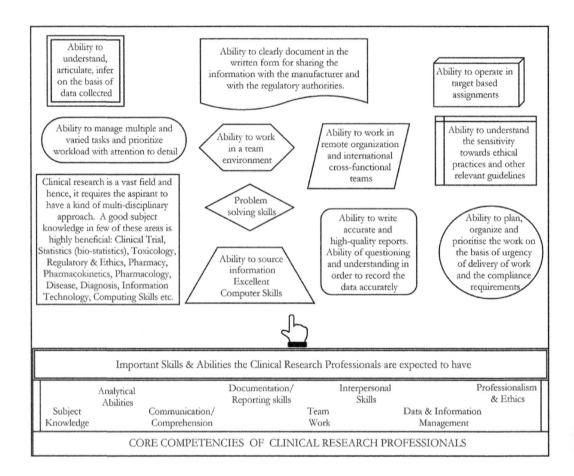

19.6 Selection Process Tips

The companies offering jobs in Clinical research field usually have a selection process in place which comprises of subject related test, aptitude tests, computer skill tests and personal interview rounds. Few common assessment areas which must be the target areas of improvement for a fresher aspiring for a job in Clinical research field are mentioned in the below table.

Assessment Areas	Purpose
Quantitative Aptitude Test	Tests the candidate's ability to deal with numbers quickly and accurately. It also tests the problem-solving ability.
Verbal Reasoning Test	Tests the ability to think constructively, accurately and quickly.

Non-Verbal (diagrammatic) Tests	Tests the logical reasoning ability and measures your ability to infer a set of rules from a flowchart or sequence of diagrams and then to apply those rules to new situation.
Situation/Scenario based Tests	Scenario based tests assess how you approach situations encountered in the workplace.
Interview – Technical Round	Tests your knowledge on the Subject
Interview (HR Round)	Tests the candidate's interpersonal skills, behavioral aspects, self-confidence, and motivation necessary for the job.
Computer Skills Tests	Tests mainly the proficiency in using MS Office Tools and internet tools apart from checking the typing accuracy.
Written - Descriptive Tests	Tests the language ability, email writing etc.

19.7 Desired personality traits of a potential candidate

A candidate is considered to be employable if he/she has the potential to be a good employee. HR round tests the candidate on employability factor mainly with regards to the personality traits of the candidate. Few such areas are mentioned in the **Fig – Desired personality traits of a potential candidate.**

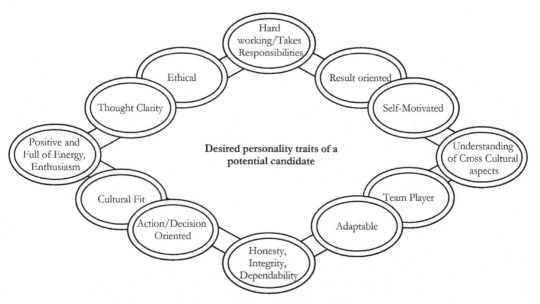

Fig: Desired personality traits of a potential candidate

19.8 Subject related questions helpful for interview preparation

- What is a clinical trial?
- What are the different types of clinical trials?
- What are the phases of clinical trials?
- What is the difference between pre-marketing and post marketing studies?
- What is the difference between adverse event and adverse drug reaction?
- What is annotated CRF?
- Why participate in a clinical trial?
- Who can participate in a clinical trial?
- What happens during a clinical trial?
- What is informed consent?
- What are the benefits and risks of participating in a clinical trial?
- What is a protocol?
- What is a placebo?
- What is the importance of Informed consent?
- How is the safety of the participant protected?
- Can a participant leave a clinical trial after it has begun?
- Where do the ideas for trials come from?
- What is the difference between a health care professional and a non-healthcare professional?
- Who are the sponsors of the clinical trials?
- What is a control group?
- Explain Clinical Research.
- Does a participant get payment for the participation in a trial?
- Is there a cost to participate in a trial?
- What is RCT?

- What are the benefits of RCT?

- What is blinding and why it is required in a clinical study?

- Define eligibility criteria.

- What is Unexpected adverse reaction and expected adverse reaction?

- List the regulatory authorities of the few countries.

- What are the timelines of SAE reporting?

- What is meant by Day Zero?

- What are the SAE criteria?

- What are the various outcomes of SAE (worst to favorable outcome)?

Chapter 20

GLOSSARY

Active Ingredient - The chemically active part of a chemical compound.

Adverse drug reaction (ADR) - ADR is an unintended reaction occurring with a drug where a positive (direct) causal relationship between the event and the drug is thought, or has been proven, to exist.

Adverse event (AE) - An AE is any untoward medical occurrence, in a patient or clinical investigation subject, administered a pharmaceutical product and that does not necessarily have a causal relationship with this treatment. An AE can therefore be any unfavourable and unintended sign (including an abnormal laboratory finding), symptom, or disease temporally associated with the use of a medicinal (investigational) product, whether or not related to the medicinal (investigational) product.

Animal model - Animal model is a living, non-human animal used during the research and investigation of human disease, for the purpose of better understanding the disease process without the added risk of harming an actual human.

Applicable regulatory requirement(s) - Any law(s) and regulation(s) addressing the conduct of clinical trials of investigational products of the jurisdiction where trial is conducted.

Approval (in relation to institutional review boards (IRBs)) - The affirmative decision of the IRB that the clinical trial has been reviewed and may be conducted at the institution site within the constraints set forth by the IRB, the institution, good clinical practice (GCP), and the applicable regulatory requirements.

Arm - Arm can be defined as any of the treatment groups in a clinical trial. Most randomized trials have two "arms," but some have three "arms," or even more.

Audit - A systematic and independent examination of trial-related activities and documents to determine whether the evaluated trial-related activities were conducted, and the data were recorded, analysed, and accurately reported according to the protocol, sponsor's standard operating procedures (SOPs), good clinical practice (GCP), and the applicable regulatory requirement(s).

Audit certificate - A declaration of confirmation by the auditor that an audit has taken place.

Audit report - A written evaluation by the sponsor's auditor of the results of the audit.

Audit trail - Documentation that allows reconstruction of the course of events.

Baseline - An initial measurement that is taken at an early time point to represent a beginning condition, and is used for comparison over time to look for changes. For example, the size of a tumour will be measured before treatment (baseline) and then afterwards to see if the treatment had an effect.

Benefit-risk profile - It is the description or analysis of whether the therapeutic benefits of using a pharmaceutical product outweigh the risks involved. This balance can be different for certain groups of patients or for those with particular coexisting conditions/diseases.

Benefits - Benefits are commonly expressed as the proven therapeutic good of a product but should also include the patient's subjective assessment of its effects.

Best practice - In medicine, treatment that experts agree is appropriate, accepted, and widely used. Health care providers are obligated to provide patients with the best practice. Also called standard therapy or standard of care.

Bias - When a point of view prevents impartial judgment on issues relating to the subject of that point of view. In clinical studies, bias is controlled by blinding and randomization.

Bioequivalence - Two pharmaceutical products are bioequivalent if they are pharmaceutically equivalent and their bioavailabilities (rate and extent of availability), after administration in the same molar dose, are similar to such a degree that their effects can be expected to be essentially the same.

Biologic - A virus, therapeutic serum, toxin, antitoxin, vaccine, blood, blood component or derivative, allergenic product, or analogous product applicable to the prevention, treatment or cure of diseases or injuries of human.

Blinding/masking - A procedure in which one or more parties to the trial are kept unaware of the treatment assignment(s). Single blinding usually refers to the subject(s) being unaware, and double blinding usually refers to the subject(s), investigator(s), monitor, and, in some cases, data analyst(s) being unaware of the treatment assignment(s).

Case report form (CRF) - A printed, optical, or electronic document designed to record all of the protocol-required information to be reported to the sponsor on each trial subject.

CRA (Clinical Research Associate) or Monitor - Person employed by the study sponsor or CRO to monitor clinical study at all participating sites and reviews study records to determine that a study is being conducted in accordance with the protocol.

Clinical Research Coordinator (CRC) - Person at clinical trial site who manages daily operations of clinical trial at site and responsible to investigator.

Clinical trial/study - Any investigation in human subjects intended to discover or verify the clinical, pharmacological, and/or other pharmacodynamic effects of an investigational product(s), and/or to identify any adverse reactions to an investigational product(s), and/or to study absorption, distribution, metabolism, and excretion of an investigational product(s) with the object of ascertaining its safety and/or efficacy. The terms clinical trial and clinical study are synonymous.

Clinical Trial/Study Report - A written description of a trial/study of any therapeutic, prophylactic, or diagnostic agent conducted in human subjects, in which the clinical and statistical description, presentations, and analyses are fully integrated into a single report.

Comparator (Product) - An investigational or marketed product (i.e., active control), or placebo, used as a reference in a clinical trial.

Compliance (in relation to trials) - Adherence to all the trial-related requirements, good clinical practice (GCP) requirements, and the applicable regulatory requirements.

Confidentiality - Prevention of disclosure, to other than authorized individuals, of a sponsor's proprietary information or of a subject's identity.

Contract - A written, dated, and signed agreement between two or more involved parties that sets out any arrangements on delegation and distribution of tasks and obligations and, if appropriate, on financial matters. The protocol may serve as the basis of a contract.

Control Group - A comparison group of study subjects who are not treated with the investigational agent. The subjects in this group may receive no therapy, a different therapy, or a placebo.

Controlled Trials - A control is a standard against which experimental observations may be evaluated. In a controlled clinical trial, one group of participants is given an experimental drug, while another group (i.e., the control group) is given either a standard treatment for the disease or a placebo.

Coordinating Committee - A committee that a sponsor may organize to coordinate the conduct of a multicentre trial.

Coordinating Investigator - An investigator assigned the responsibility for the coordination of investigators at different centres participating in a multicentre trial.

Contract Research Organization (CRO) - A person or an organization (commercial, academic, or other) contracted by the sponsor to perform one or more of a sponsor's trial-related duties and functions.

Crossover Trial - A clinical trial in which all participants receive both treatments, but at different times. At a predetermined point in the study, one group is switched from the experimental treatment to the control treatment (standard treatment), and the other group is switched from the control to the experimental treatment.

Direct Access - Permission to examine, analyse, verify, and reproduce any records and reports that are important to evaluation of a clinical trial. Any party (e.g., domestic and foreign regulatory authorities, sponsors, monitors, and auditors) with direct access should take all reasonable precautions within the constraints of the applicable regulatory requirement(s) to maintain the confidentiality of subjects' identities and sponsor's proprietary information.

Documentation - All records, in any form (including, but not limited to, written, electronic, magnetic, and optical records; and scans, x-rays, and electrocardiograms) that describe or record the methods, conduct, and/or results of a trial, the factors affecting a trial, and the actions taken.

Endpoint - Overall outcome that the protocol is designed to evaluate.

Enrolling - The act of signing up participants into a study. Generally, this process involves evaluating a participant with respect to the eligibility criteria of the study and going through the informed consent process.

Essential Documents - Documents that individually and collectively permit evaluation of the conduct of a study and the quality of the data produced.

Eligibility Criteria - Summary of criteria for participant selection; includes inclusion and exclusion criteria.

Exclusion /Inclusion criteria - There are characteristics that must be present (inclusion) or absent (exclusion) in order for a subject to qualify for a trial as per the protocol of the trial.

Experimental Drug(product) - A drug that is not FDA licensed for use in humans, or as a treatment for a particular condition.

Experimental group - The group of subjects exposed to the new, researched treatment. This group is often compared to a 'control group' (the subjects who are not exposed to that treatment).

Good Clinical Practice (GCP) - A standard for the design, conduct, performance, monitoring, auditing, recording, analyses, and reporting of clinical trials that provides assurance that the data and reported results are credible and accurate, and that the rights, integrity, and confidentiality of trial subjects are protected.

Independent Data Monitoring Committee (IDMC) (Data and Safety Monitoring Board, Monitoring Committee, Data Monitoring Committee) - An independent data monitoring committee that may be established by the sponsor to assess at intervals the progress of a clinical trial, the safety data, and the critical efficacy endpoints, and to recommend to the sponsor whether to continue, modify, or stop a trial.

Impartial Witness - A person, who is independent of the trial, who cannot be unfairly influenced by people involved with the trial, who attends the informed consent process if the subject or the subject's legally acceptable representative cannot read, and who reads the informed consent form and any other written information supplied to the subject.

Independent Ethics Committee (IEC) - An independent group of both medical and non-medical professionals who are responsible for verifying the integrity of a study and ensuring the safety, integrity, and human rights of the study participants.

Indication - A symptom that suggests certain medical treatment is necessary.

Informed Consent - A process by which a subject voluntarily confirms his or her willingness to participate in a particular trial, after having been informed of all aspects of the trial that are relevant to the subject's decision to participate. Informed consent is documented by means of a written, signed, and dated informed consent form.

Informed Consent Document - A document explaining all relevant study information to assist the study volunteer in understanding the expectations and requirements of participation in a clinical trial. This document is presented to and signed by the study subject.

Inpatient - A patient who lives in hospital while under treatment.

Inspection - The act by a regulatory authority(ies) of conducting an official review of documents, facilities, records, and any other resources that are deemed by the authority(ies) to be related to the clinical trial and that may be located at the site of the trial, at the sponsor's and/or contract research organization's (CROs) facilities, or at other establishments deemed appropriate by the regulatory authority(ies).

Institution (medical) - Any public or private entity or agency or medical or dental facility where clinical trials are conducted.

Institutional Review Board (IRB) - An independent group of professionals designated to review and approve the clinical protocol, informed consent forms, study advertisements, and patient brochures, to ensure that the study is safe and effective for human participation. It is also the IRB's responsibility to ensure that the study adheres to the FDA's regulations.

Interim Clinical Trial/Study Report - A report of intermediate results and their evaluation based on analyses performed during the course of a trial.

Investigational Product - A pharmaceutical form of an active ingredient or placebo being tested or used as a reference in a clinical trial, including a product with a marketing authorization when used or assembled (formulated or packaged) in a way different from the approved form, or when used for an unapproved indication, or when used to gain further information about an approved use.

Investigator - A person responsible for the conduct of the clinical trial at a trial site. If a trial is conducted by a team of individuals at a trial site, the investigator is the responsible leader of the team and may be called the principal investigator.

Investigator's Brochure - A compilation of the clinical and nonclinical data on the investigational product(s) that is relevant to the study of the investigational product(s) in human subjects.

Legally Acceptable Representative - An individual or juridical or other body authorized under applicable law to consent, on behalf of a prospective subject, to the subject's participation in the clinical trial.

MAH (Marketing Authorization holder) - MAH is usually an organization to whom permission has been granted for marketing the medicinal product (s) for specified indication.

Manufacturer - A person or company that makes products/goods for sale.

Marketing authorization - An official document issued by the competent drug regulatory authority for the purpose of marketing or free distribution of a product after evaluation for safety, efficacy and quality.

Medical History - A narrative or record of past events and circumstances that are or may be relevant to a patient's current state of health. Informally, an account of past diseases, injuries, treatments, and other strictly medical facts.

Monitoring - The act of overseeing the progress of a clinical trial, and of ensuring that it is conducted, recorded, and reported in accordance with the protocol, standard operating procedures (SOPs), GCP, and the applicable regulatory requirement(s).

Monitoring Report - A written report from the monitor to the sponsor after each site visit and/or other trial-related communication according to the sponsor's SOPs.

Multicentre Trial - A clinical trial conducted according to a single protocol but at more than one site, and, therefore, carried out by more than one investigator.

Nonclinical Study - Biomedical studies not performed on human subjects.

Open-Label Trial - A clinical trial in which doctors and participants know which treatment is being administered.

Opinion (in relation to Independent Ethics Committee) - The judgment and/or the advice provided by an Independent Ethics Committee (IEC).

Original Medical Record - See Source Documents.

Outpatient - A patient who visits a health care facility for diagnosis or treatment without spending the night, sometimes called a day patient.

Parallel trial(study) - A parallel designed clinical trial compares the results of a treatment on two separate groups of patients. The sample size calculated for a parallel design can be used for any study where two groups are being compared.

Pre-marketing - The stage before a drug is available for prescription or sale to the public.

Principal Investigator - A person responsible for the overall conduct of the clinical trial at a trial site. If a trial is conducted by a team of individuals at a trial site, the investigator is the responsible leader of the team and may be called the principal investigator.

Protocol - A document that describes the objective(s), design, methodology, statistical considerations, and organization of a trial. The protocol usually also gives the background and rationale for the trial, but these could be provided in other protocol referenced documents.

Protocol Amendment - A written description of a change(s) to or formal clarification of a protocol.

Placebo -A placebo is an inactive pill, liquid, or powder that has no treatment value. In clinical trials, experimental treatments are often compared with placebos to assess the treatment's effectiveness.

Placebo Controlled Trial - A method of drug investigation in which an inactive substance (a placebo) is given to one group of participants, while the drug being tested is given to another group. The results obtained in the two groups are then compared to see if the investigational treatment is more effective than the placebo in treating the condition.

Placebo Effect - A physical or emotional change, occurring after an inactive substance is taken or administered, that is not the result of any special property of the substance. The change may be beneficial, reflecting the expectations of the participant and, often, the expectations of the person giving the substance.

Post-marketing - The stage when a drug is generally available on the market.

Quality Assurance (QA) - All those planned and systematic actions that are established to ensure that the trial is performed and the data are generated, documented (recorded), and reported in compliance with GCP and the applicable regulatory requirement(s).

Quality Control (QC) - The operational techniques and activities undertaken within the quality assurance system to verify that the requirements for quality of the trial related activities have been fulfilled.

Randomization - The process of assigning trial subjects to treatment or control groups using an element of chance to determine the assignments in order to reduce bias.

Randomized Trial - A study in which participants are randomly (i.e., by chance) assigned to one of two or more treatment arms of a clinical trial.

Regulatory Authorities - Bodies having the power to regulate. In the ICH GCP guidance, the expression "Regulatory Authorities" includes the authorities that review submitted clinical data and those that conduct inspections. These bodies are sometimes referred to as competent authorities.

Risk - The probability that an event will occur.

Risk factors - Risk factors are any attribute, characteristic or exposure of an individual that increases the likelihood of developing a disease or injury.

Safety - Relative freedom from harm

Sample Size - A subset of a larger population, selected for investigation to draw conclusions or make estimates about the larger population.

Serious Adverse Event (SAE) or Serious Adverse Drug Reaction (Serious ADR) - Any untoward medical occurrence that at any dose:

- Results in death,

- Is life-threatening,

- Requires inpatient hospitalization or prolongation of existing hospitalization,

- Results in persistent or significant disability/incapacity, or

- Is a congenital anomaly/birth defect

- Is important medical event

Source Data - All information in original records and certified copies of original records of clinical findings, observations, or other activities in a clinical trial necessary for the reconstruction and evaluation of the trial. Source data are contained in source documents (original records or certified copies).

Source Documents - Original documents, data, and records (e.g., hospital records, clinical and office charts, laboratory notes, memoranda, subjects' diaries or evaluation checklists, pharmacy dispensing records, recorded data from automated instruments, copies or transcriptions certified after verification as being accurate and complete, microfiches, photographic negatives, microfilm or magnetic media, x-rays, subject files, and records kept at the pharmacy, at the laboratories, and at medico-technical departments involved in the clinical trial).

Sponsor - An individual, company, institution, or organization that takes responsibility for the initiation, management, and/or financing of a clinical trial.

Sponsor-Investigator - An individual who both initiates and conducts, alone or with others, a clinical trial, and under whose immediate direction the investigational product is administered to, dispensed to, or used by a subject. The term does not include any person other than an individual (e.g., it does not include a corporation or an agency). The obligations of a sponsor-investigator include both those of a sponsor and those of an investigator.

Standard Operating Procedures (SOPs) - Detailed, written instructions to achieve uniformity of the performance of a specific function.

Sub investigator - Any individual member of the clinical trial team designated and supervised by the investigator at a trial site to perform critical trial-related procedures and/or to make important trial-related decisions (e.g., associates, residents, research fellows).

Subject/Trial Subject - An individual who participates in a clinical trial, either as a recipient of the investigational product(s) or as a control.

Subject Identification Code - A unique identifier assigned by the investigator to each trial subject to protect the subject's identity and used in lieu of the subject's name when the investigator reports adverse events and/or other trial-related data.

Trial Site - The location(s) where trial-related activities are actually conducted.

Unexpected Adverse Drug Reaction - An adverse reaction, the nature or severity of which is not consistent with the applicable product information (e.g., Investigator's Brochure for an unapproved investigational product or package insert/summary of product characteristics for an approved product).

Vulnerable Subjects - Individuals whose willingness to volunteer in a clinical trial may be unduly influenced by the expectation, whether justified or not, of benefits associated with participation, or of a retaliatory response from senior members of a hierarchy in case of refusal to participate. Examples are members of a group with a hierarchical structure, such as medical, pharmacy, dental, and nursing students, subordinate hospital and laboratory personnel, employees of the pharmaceutical industry, members of the armed forces, and persons kept in detention. Other vulnerable subjects include patients with incurable diseases, persons in nursing homes, unemployed or impoverished persons, patients in emergency situations, ethnic minority groups, homeless persons, nomads, refugees, minors, and those incapable of giving consent.

Well-being (of the trial subjects) - The physical and mental integrity of the subjects participating in a clinical trial.

Printed in Great Britain
by Amazon